The Good Mentoring Toolkit for Healthcare

Helen Bayley

Facilitator
Shropshire and Staffordshire Clinical Leadership Programme

Ruth Chambers

General Practitioner
Clinical Dean
Staffordshire University
Head of Stoke-on-Trent Teaching PCT Programme

and

Caroline Donovan

Head of Learning, Education and Training
Shropshire PCTs

Radcliffe Publishing Ltd
18 Marcham Road
Abingdon
Oxon OX14 1AA
United Kingdom

www.radcliffe-oxford.com
Electronic catalogue and worldwide online ordering facility.

Reprinted 2006

British Library Cataloguing in Publication Data

A catalogue record for this book is available from the British Library.

ISBN 1 85775 649 5

Typeset by Advance Typesetting Ltd, Oxfordshire
Printed and bound by TJI Digital, Padstow, Cornwall

Contents

About the authors

Helen Bayley is a facilitator with the Shropshire and Staffordshire Clinical Leadership Programme. Promoting effective mentoring relationships on the clinical leadership programme and leadership at the point of care programme are an integral part of her role. She also facilitates mentoring workshops for other professionals across organisations within Shropshire and Staffordshire. Helen is a nurse by background and had previously been a ward sister for seven years on an adult acute medical ward. It was while working in an intensive care unit that Helen experienced her first successful mentoring relationship and she has since been mentored by nurses, managers and physicians. Mentoring has been of vital support to her over the years, and she firmly believes that it is key to meeting the NHS modernisation agenda. Through both her positive and negative experiences of being a mentee and mentor, Helen is keen to help others to gain the support they need in meeting the demands on them within a clinical setting in today's stressful climate.

Ruth Chambers has been a GP for more than 20 years. Her previous experience has encompassed a wide range of research and educational activities, with a focus on stress and the health of doctors, the quality of healthcare, healthy working, teenagers' contraception and many other topics.

She is currently a part-time GP, Head of Stoke-on-Trent Teaching Primary Care Trust programme and the Professor of Primary Care Development at Staffordshire University. Ruth has established a mentoring scheme for doctors working in primary care in North Staffordshire to aid their retention and development. She has worked with the Kent, Surrey and Sussex Deanery to develop a job description of a mentor based on the NHS Knowledge and Skills Framework, which is described in this book.

Caroline Donovan is a nurse and health visitor by background. Her previous experience has been in health promotion, education and general management. More recently she has developed multidisciplinary leadership programmes across Shropshire and Staffordshire health and social care organisations. Her current role is as Head of Learning, Education and Training across the Primary Care Trusts in Shropshire.

Caroline has established and developed mentoring as an integral element of leadership programmes and believes that mentoring has enormous potential for the development of future leaders across the healthcare community. To date, more than 800 mentors and mentees have been supported in their leadership development within the NHS throughout Shropshire and Staffordshire.

Acknowledgements

We should like to acknowledge the contributions and support from Abdol Tavabie, Gill Wakley, Kay Mohanna, Wendy Garcarz, Anthony Schwartz, Rachel Brown and Lynn Turner. In particular, we should like to thank Rachel, a Changing Working Practice facilitator, for her contribution of *The Three Brains, Be Your Own Hero* and *The Rucksack* exercises, which she amended from the BBC Conference Lab for use in the Shropshire and Staffordshire Clinical Leadership Facilitators toolkit.[1] Gill and Kay have co-authored a considerable amount of material with Ruth, from which some of the tools and techniques were derived. Gill has worked with Ruth to devise the 5-stage cycle of evidence to demonstrate competency.[2,3] Abdol has worked with Ruth and others in Kent, Surrey and Sussex Deanery to develop a template for a competency-based job description for mentors using the NHS Knowledge and Skills Framework.[4,5] Wendy has contributed documentation from the mentoring scheme she set up with Ruth at Stoke-on-Trent Teaching Primary Care Trust, with funding from West Midlands Deanery.[6] Anthony has agreed that documentation developed by Arcadia Alive may be included too.

The Good Mentoring Toolkit for Healthcare shares similar resource materials to those included in *The Good Appraisal Toolkit for Primary Care*[7] with respect to a mentor's competence in the core and specific Dimensions of the NHS Knowledge and Skills Framework.[5]

References

1 Shropshire and Staffordshire Clinical Leadership Team (2002) *Clinical Leadership Facilitators Handbook.* Shropshire and Staffordshire Strategic Health Authority, Telford.

2 Chambers R, Wakley G, Field S and Ellis S (2002) *Appraisal for the Apprehensive.* Radcliffe Medical Press, Oxford.

3 Chambers R, Mohanna K, Wakley G and Wall D (2004) *Demonstrating Your Competency as a Healthcare Teacher.* Radcliffe Medical Press, Oxford.

4 Chambers R, Tavabie A, See S and Hughes S (2004) Template for a competency based job description for mentors using the NHS Knowledge and Skills Framework. *Education for Primary Care.* **15**: 220–30.

5 Department of Health (2003) *The NHS Knowledge and Skills Framework. Version 6.* Department of Health, London.

6 Garcarz W (2004) *Effective Mentoring for Mentors.* 4 Health Ltd, Birmingham. www.4-health.biz

7 Chambers R, Tavabie A, Mohanna K and Wakley G (2004) *The Good Appraisal Toolkit for Primary Care.* Radcliffe Publishing, Oxford and San Francisco.

Introduction

This toolkit can be used to help you establish good practice in mentoring, whether you are being mentored, an individual mentor, or responsible for setting up a mentoring scheme in your organisation – hospital or primary care trust, deanery, college, etc. It will guide you as to what to expect from mentoring and provide practical help in setting up the components of a mentoring scheme. Chapter 1 includes the many and varied definitions of mentoring. We employ general definitions of mentoring throughout this toolkit, rather than employing any terminology specific to one professional group. In brief, the benefits of mentoring for individuals are:

- increases the confidence of the mentee[1] by:
  - supporting them while they learn new skills, behaviours, etc.
  - challenging assumptions
  - offering alternative perspectives
  - facilitating the mentee in finding solutions to their problems
- encourages reflective practice by:
  - providing a sounding board
  - providing protected time and space to consider professional practice
  - increasing mentees' understanding of their working environment
- enhances self-development through:
  - action planning and learning
  - effective goal setting
  - increasing professional confidence and professional credibility.

Successive chapters will guide you in setting up mentoring to pursue these benefits for individuals taking part. In Chapter 2, we consider the gains from all perspectives – the mentee, the mentor, an employing organisation and the NHS in general – for informal mentoring relationships and formal mentoring schemes.

Chapters 3 and 4 present tools and techniques that a mentor might adopt to improve their knowledge and skills. These are based on the dimensions of the NHS Knowledge and Skills Framework, part of the Agenda for Change initiative,[2] which are relevant to a mentor's role and responsibilities. Chapter 5 provides a five-staged approach for mentors to consider using as a way of gathering evidence to demonstrate that they are competent. This model can be generalised to all other aspects of a mentor's work – whether they have a clinical, managerial or support post in the NHS.

Chapter 6 gives useful tips and practical tools to allow the mentee to take advantage of the mentoring relationship – and to capitalise on their strengths and opportunities, and address any weaknesses.

There are activities interspersed throughout the toolkit, which should help you to check out how competent you are or reinforce your personal and professional development or learning – from mentor, mentee or scheme perspectives. Mentors may recommend an activity to a mentee for their own development or they may work through it together.

Finally, in Chapter 7, we supply all the documentation you will require as mentors or mentees to draw up your contract or use to define your roles or set up the mentoring scheme in your organisation or workplace.

e-learning option

There is great scope for using existing training materials in more innovative ways, such as via e-learning or electronic distribution. Evidence suggests that levels of computer literacy do not need to be high to use e-learning materials, and that healthcare professionals actually prefer to learn at home, believing it is a method that helps to address their work–life balance issues.[3]

The Shropshire and Staffordshire Clinical Leadership Team are currently building on their existing mentoring work to allow a huge expansion in the mentoring aspect of their programme. Their 'mentoring toolkit' has been converted into an electronic form with an interactive workbook that will be accessible via the website www. telfordpct.com. E-learning will be offered alongside the existing programme in order to:

- further develop the evidence base
- help manage problems of releasing clinical staff
- provide a cost-effective way of continuing to train and develop staff after completion of the programme
- allow access from home or work
- enable material to be repeated to ensconce learning
- fit with programme participants' work–life balance.

All electronic work is being prepared in conjunction with David Dawes at the European Nursing Leadership Foundation.[3]

References

1 Garcarz W (2004) *Effective Mentoring for Mentors.* 4 Health Ltd, Birmingham. www.4-health.biz

2 Department of Health (2003) *The NHS Knowledge and Skills Framework. Version 6.* Department of Health, London.

3 The European Nursing Leadership Foundation, 308 Ducie House, Ducie Street, Manchester www.nursingleadership.org.uk

1

What is mentoring?

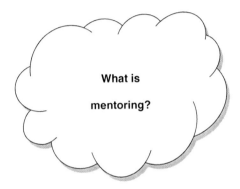

What is

mentoring?

An organisation which offers structured mentorship is an organisation with more fulfilled, committed, resourceful and motivated employees, who will stay within that organisation.

Cunningham[1]

Mentoring in healthcare settings

Mentoring has existed for thousands of years in a variety of cultures. The word 'mentor' originates from Greek mythology and the story of Odysseus, who, when setting off on his journey to Troy, entrusted his friend Mentor with the care and education of his son Telemachus. Legend has it that Odysseus instructed Mentor to 'Tell him all that you know', unwittingly setting the standard for aspiring mentors.

Mentoring is a transformational process that seeks to help individuals develop and use knowledge to improve themselves on an ongoing basis. It is a professional dialogue that encourages reflection and development, signposting mentees to other sources of help as required.

A review of mentoring in relation to general medical practice described mentoring as 'a way of helping another understand more fully, and learn comprehensively from, their day to day experience'.[2] An enquiry into mentoring commissioned by the Department of Health defined mentoring as a 'process whereby an experienced, highly regarded, empathic person (the mentor), guides another individual (the mentee) in the development and re-examination of their own ideas, learning, and personal and professional development. The mentor, who often, but not necessarily works in the same organisation or field as the mentee, achieves this by listening and talking in confidence to the mentee.'[3] This definition was derived from work relating to medical, dental and other healthcare professions and general management.

Another definition of mentoring by Carmin, derived in an organisational context rather than applying specifically to a health setting, considered mentoring to be a 'complex, interactive process occurring between individuals of differing levels of experience and expertise which incorporates interpersonal or psychosocial development, and socialisation functions into the relationship. This one-to-one relationship is itself developmental and proceeds through a series of stages which help to determine both the conditions affecting, and the outcomes of, the process. To the extent that the parameters of mutuality and compatibility exist in the relationship, the potential outcomes of respect, professionalism, collegiality and role fulfilment will result. Further, the mentoring process occurs in a dynamic relationship within a given milieu.'[4]

Box 1.1: What is mentoring? Other general definitions

'Helping another person become what that person aspires to'[5]

'Mentoring is a powerful form of management learning, in which an experienced individual passes on know-how to someone less experienced'[6]

'The mentor represents knowledge, reflection, insight, understanding, good advice, determination and planning, qualities that cannot be mastered alone'[7]

'Off-line help by one person to another in making significant transitions, in knowledge, working or thinking'[1]

The definitions of mentoring from the health setting[2,3,5] that we have included so far are similar to those describing the process in organisations as a whole.[4,6,7] But in nursing and midwifery the term 'mentor' can be used specifically to denote the role of the nurse, midwife or health visitor who facilitates learning and supervises and assesses students in the practice setting – as given in Box 1.2.[8,9,10] We will be using the general definitions of mentoring and mentor throughout this toolkit, rather than employing any terminology specific to one professional group.

Box 1.2: Role of mentor from student nurse's perspective[8,9,10]

(i) Supporter: give nurse advice, sort out problems or worries, be there as ally or friend
(ii) Guide and teacher: explain things, organise and arrange visits, be role model, feedback on performance to nurse
(iii) Supervisor: share problems, talk about mistakes and uncertainties, enable nurse to work out own solutions, allow gradual independence
(iv) Assessor: good understanding of assessment process and outcomes, implement assessment procedures

What's in it for you?

With increasing pressures on everyone's working day in the NHS, it is vital to find new ways of coping and thriving at work. Mentoring supports professionals' growth in knowledge, skills, attributes and practice.

If you have a mentor, your mentoring relationship will provide you with the confidential opportunity to share your feelings, express your views, test out ideas and raise questions. It will allow you to take a step back and look at yourself, as a manager, as a leader, as a health professional or team player and most importantly at you as a person.

You will be asking yourself soul-searching questions: Where are you at in your career? Where do you want to be? How can you get there? Who can help you to get there? If you are happy where you are, you will be considering:

* What makes you feel fulfilled at work?
* What aspects of your practice would you like to capitalise on?
* What aspects of your work or practice would you like to develop?
* How can you maintain job satisfaction over time?

How can you expect to lead others efficiently if you are unable to accept your own strengths and weaknesses? How can you expect to lead others efficiently if you are feeling burnt out yourself? How can you expect to lead others efficiently if you do not allow yourself time out to look at how you do things and why you do them that way?

If you are a mentor, you will benefit from gaining more insights into how you work and act, as you challenge the thinking and perceptions of your mentee(s). You will gain considerable self-satisfaction too from helping others, which will probably boost your own job satisfaction and make you more aware of your work environment.

How does mentoring fit with the NHS agenda?

The NHS Plan (2000) requires a fundamental change in thinking, practice and the delivery of healthcare over the next decade.[11] The Plan's ambitious agenda is challenging. We know that managers and health and social care professionals can meet these challenges to improve services by learning from each other and basing their decisions on evidence from research literature and evaluation when possible.

The NHS Plan supports continuing professional development (CPD) to deliver patient-focused healthcare. In addition, the Department of Health's *Working Together – Learning Together* document[12] emphasises that lifelong learning and development are key to delivering the government's vision of patient/client-focused care within the NHS.

Another Department of Health document, *Managing for Excellence in the NHS*,[13] indicates that we need to build on good relationships in the NHS and with our partner organisations to create a more participative and open culture where everyone can contribute. This culture needs to be creative, challenging and supportive to the workforce. It needs to embrace modern ways of working through teams and networks rather than through hierarchies and formal systems. It needs to recognise the complexity of the healthcare environment and the work that we do.

In addition, we must lead change as well as manage it. We need leadership in setting out the vision and working with and through people to achieve it. The NHS is made up of many different staff groups and supported by many different organisations. There are strong professional organisations and affiliations. There are important partnerships with social services, education, other parts of local government and the public sector, patient groups and voluntary organisations, and, increasingly, with the private sector. Mentoring is key to all of this.

All of these groups and organisations need to be involved and enabled to contribute to the transformation of the NHS. Together they can build a momentum for change – a coalition for improvement.[13]

Fostering a mentoring relationship develops, supports and equips staff with the skills they need to:

- support changes and improvements in patient care
- take advantage of wider care opportunities
- realise their potential.

The report in Box 1.3 gives the perspectives of senior executives in one health authority on the importance of the NHS investing in mentoring for its workforce.[14]

Box 1.3: Report of perceptions about mentoring in one health authority[14]

There can be a perception that mentoring is not for senior people, but for people lower down the organisation – but it can help everyone. There is a need to make it legitimate – something that represents a worthwhile investment in people, for more senior people to feel comfortable in having and using mentors.

Where the culture is not supportive, mentoring is threatening and not productive if the mentors work in the same organisation as the mentees. If mentoring is to benefit the performance of the organisation through the wellbeing and high quality of performance of its staff, then the blockages need to be identified and removed or ameliorated.

Senior executives suggested:

- awareness raising of benefits of mentoring: role models, case studies, links to workshops on changing roles, conferences
- make mentoring legitimate – 'coming out of the closet', taking away the perception that mentoring is a remedial activity
- encourage mentoring to be seen as an investment in people
- identify and communicate who is willing to do what – so that there is less secrecy
- make mentoring one aspect of management development
- mentoring should not be compulsory.

How does mentoring benefit individuals?[15,16]

You may not agree with all our suggestions listed below, depending on your experience and perspective of mentoring. These have been collated from the various reports of mentoring cited earlier in this chapter. Mentoring is a developmental process for the mentee who should gain from:

- improved performance that can be evaluated back in the workplace and lead to more defined objectives at the next mentoring session
- new insights and perspectives from another individual's or professional's point of view
- increased confidence and self-knowledge

- better interpersonal skills
- an increase in personal influencing skills
- knowledge and skills, including technical skills
- having their perceptions and beliefs challenged
- enjoying the challenges of change
- an open and flexible attitude to learning
- overcoming setbacks and obstacles
- developing values and an ethical perspective
- increasing listening, analytical and problem-solving skills
- conscious reflection that enhances learning
- career development
- learning opportunities
- dispassionate feedback from another person
- advice and skills in relation to handling people
- personal growth
- specific help with new tasks
- some degree of sponsorship and recommendation from mentor
- 'political' knowledge and access to informal network of mentor.

One review of the benefits of mentoring for doctors logged many examples of changes made as a result of mentoring, as described in Box 1.4.

Box 1.4: Outcomes of mentoring for individual doctors reported in a review[17]

1 Helped with serious problems encountered in their professional lives
2 Regaining personal and professional confidence that had been undermined by a feeling of loss of control over their professional lives and an accompanying sense that their competence was at risk. The experience of mentoring had given individuals confidence to, for example:
- take control
- take action on matters that had previously been 'pending'
- manage complex job responsibilities
- deal with difficult relationships
- be themselves
- remain in the profession
- leave the profession
- extend their professional roles and activities

3 Other achievements ranged over:
- increased job satisfaction
- being skilled helper
- improved working relationships with colleagues
- helped to identify the core of the problem
- understood underlying issues
- developed new ways to approach and manage problems
- come to understand problems in different and sometimes surprising ways
- associated with an increased feeling of wellbeing
- increased confidence in leadership role
- greater understanding of the perspectives of others
- identified educational needs
- made career choices
- clarified a sense of professional identity and purpose

What distinguishes a mentor from other supportive roles?

Table 1.1 distinguishes some of the most commonly used roles that professionals may adopt as part of providing personal and professional development and support to staff. There is often confusion over what differentiates the terms and descriptions from each other.

Table 1.1:   Differentiating the term mentor from other roles

Role	One to one	Group	Long-term	Short-term	Management-led	Personal development	Professional development
Coach	X			X		X	X
Mentor	X		X			X	X
Preceptor	X			X			X
Assessor	X			X	X		X
Clinical supervisor	X	X	X			X	X
Appraiser	X			X	X		X

You might be a mentor, coach, supervisor, assessor or appraiser to several people, or more than one of these to the same person. There are many overlaps between all these terms but the differences in the role of each are distinct. The terms are all part of common parlance and those in authority may believe that people have the skills for a particular role by virtue of their position, not understanding the specific roles and responsibilities of being a good supervisor, trainer, mentor or careers counsellor, etc. Sometimes one individual is expected to be a mentor, educational supervisor, line manager and careers counsellor to the same person and conflicts of interest can arise. For example, it is difficult for everyone involved if someone acting as the careers counsellor has authority over the member of staff and the ability to change their work circumstances in a negative way, as the individual is unlikely to trust in the independence of the careers counsellor, and the careers counsellor may act on their acquired insider knowledge on a future occasion.

Some of the other roles can be described as follows.

A careers counsellor acts to help people:

- understand their emotions, abilities, interests and special aptitudes
- make and carry out appropriate life choices and plans, and achieve satisfactory adjustments in life
- acquire information about educational and career opportunities within a changing society.

A coach[18] motivates, encourages and helps an individual to improve their skills, knowledge and attitudes in their personal and professional lives so that the person:

- is challenged to perform at their best

- deepens their learning
- enhances their quality of life
- focuses on specific objectives within a defined time period.

A preceptor[19] is an experienced individual who provides clinical and professional support to facilitate student learning:

- usually short term
- to enable individuals to develop knowledge and competence after someone has recently qualified, or when someone needs to learn a specific skill
- by supervising, teaching, role modelling and evaluating students – orientating the student to the role at work and monitoring progress.

Preceptorship is usually more intensive than clinical supervision.

A clinical supervisor is an experienced person who supports an individual or group in either the short or long term and:

- aims to develop knowledge and competence, encourage self-assessment, and analytical and reflective skills
- enhances consumer protection and safety of care in complex clinical situations.

An appraiser (as the term is used in the NHS[20]) conducts a professional conversation with another person and gives them constructive feedback about their performance in relation to personal and organisational goals, on behalf of an employing organisation. They may provide assistance in progression to those goals.

An assessor[20] conducts an assessment on another individual to identify the presence or absence of quality standards. This may involve a judgemental or value-free ascertainment of the extent to which standards have been attained by the individual.

As a mentor, your relationship with your mentee should be one of mutual trust and respect in a supportive yet challenging relationship. You should not be put in the position of undertaking assessments or appraisals of a mentee, as this may undermine your relationship and create a conflict of interest. This will preclude you from being non-judgemental as a mentor, which is a cornerstone of mentoring.

References

1 Cunningham I (2001) *Mentoring; its role in changing the organisation culture.* Centre for Self-Managed Learning, Middlesex University, Middlesex.

2 Freeman R (1998) *Mentoring in General Practice.* Butterworth-Heinemann, Woburn.

3 Standing Committee on Postgraduate Medical and Dental Education (SCOPME) (1998) *Supporting Doctors and Dentists at Work. An Enquiry into Mentoring.* SCOPME, London.

4 Carmin CN (1988) Issues on research in mentoring: definitional and methodological. *International Journal of Mentoring.* **2**: 9–13.

5 NHS Leadership Programme for Chief Executives (2000) Mentoring Programme for Chief Executives. Unpublished.

6 Clutterbuck D (1993) *A Guide to Mentoring.* Clutterbuck Associates and Oxford Regional Health Authority, Oxford.

7 East A (1995) *Making Sense of Managing Culture.* Thompson Business Press, Oxford.

8 English National Board for Nursing, Midwifery and Health Visiting and Department of Health (2001) *Preparation of Mentors and Teachers.* ENB, London.

9 Gray MA and Smith LN (2000) The qualities of an effective mentor from the student nurse's perspective: findings from a longitudinal qualitative study. *J Adv Nurs.* **32**: 1542–9.

10 Gould D, Kelly D and Gouldstone L (2001) Preparing nurse managers to mentor students. *Nursing Standard.* **16(11)**: 39–42.

11 Department of Health (2000) *The NHS Plan.* Department of Health, London.

12 Department of Health (2001) *Working Together – Learning Together.* Department of Health, London.

13 Department of Health (2002) *Managing for Excellence in the NHS.* Department of Health, London.

14 Matthews F, Evans L and Garside M (1993) *A Project to Develop Guidance on Mentoring for Senior Executives.* Yorkshire Regional Health Authority, Leeds.

15 Garcarz W (2003) *Effective Mentoring for Clinicians. Stoke-on-Trent Teaching PCT.* 4 Health Ltd, Birmingham.

16 Mohanna K, Wall D and Chambers R (2003) *Teaching Made Easy. A Manual for Health Professionals* (2e). Radcliffe Medical Press, Oxford.

17 Oxley J, Fleming B, Golding L *et al.* (2003) *Mentoring for Doctors: enhancing the benefit.* Improving Working Lives for Doctors, Doctors' Forum, Department of Health, London.

18 Kersley S (2004) The ABC of change. *BMJ Careers.* **328**: s47.

19 Sachdeva AK (1996) Preceptorship, mentorship and the adult learner in medical and health sciences education. *J Cancer Educ.* **11**: 131–6.

20 Chambers R, Tavabie A, Mohanna K and Wakley G (2004) *The Good Appraisal Toolkit for Primary Care.* Radcliffe Publishing, Oxford and San Francisco.

2

Making the most of mentoring

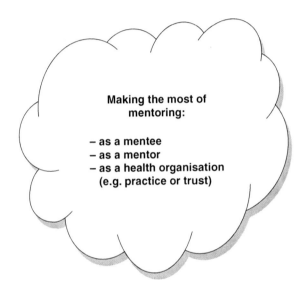

Making the most of
mentoring:

– as a mentee
– as a mentor
– as a health organisation
(e.g. practice or trust)

The mentee's perspective

When first embarking on establishing a mentoring relationship, it is important that there is openness and honesty between the employer or line manager, the mentee and the mentor. If the employer or line manager is going to support the time out for mentoring, they should be aware of the benefits and not feel that mentoring poses any threat, e.g. from a newly empowered member of staff. The benefits from having a mentor will soon emerge to all involved, in the form of greater commitment, enthusiasm and learning on the part of the mentees.

If you are seeking a mentor, there may be a formal mentoring system within your organisation where a mentor is assigned to you. Consider the list of reasons in Box 2.1 as to why you might seek a mentor, and if you believe the choice of your mentor (whether they were selected for you or you picked them yourself) is inappropriate then do not be afraid to challenge the system and find a mentor whom you think will be more suitable.

Box 2.1:   Why have a mentor?

1   Enables mutual development:
   • stepping stone to other opportunities
   • opportunities for learning: encourages your greater understanding and deeper insights
   • helps to address problems with relationships with colleagues at work
2   Increases confidence over time:
   • supports you
   • challenges: helps you to justify your chosen course of action
   • offers you alternative perspectives
   • helps you to take control, e.g. of aspects of your work or career development
   • aids you in managing complex job responsibilities
3   Encourages reflective practice – your mentor can:
   • act as a 'sounding board'
   • provide protected time and space for you to discuss issues and reflect on action
   • increase your understanding of your own environment, and the influences on your performance
   • enable you to solve problems – new approaches to solving problems, coming to understand problems in different ways
4   Enhances self-development:
   • through action planning and learning
   • through goal setting: creating your learning contract, visualising your achievements
   • develops your professional confidence
   • enhances your professional credibility
   • increased confidence in your leadership role and gives you a greater understanding of the perspectives of others
5   Increases job satisfaction

Activity 2.1: (for mentees)

What does mentoring mean to you? Have a go at describing the meaning below:
   •

   •

   •

   •

   •

Activity 2.2: (for mentees)

Why would you benefit from having a mentor? Consider how a mentor might support you in your self-development and in your day-to-day work. List the key areas below:

-

-

-

-

-

What qualities might you look for in a mentor?

The suggested lists of essential and desirable attributes given in Box 2.2 have been derived from a variety of sources. Some of these qualities will be more important to you than others. There may be other qualities that are really important to you that you will want to add, maybe relating to gender, age, type of background or experience.

Box 2.2: Qualities of a mentor

Essential	*Desirable*
Impartial	Knowledge
Good listener	Technical expertise
Supportive	Instructor
Interested	Authority
Perceptive	Advisor
Self-aware	Seniority
Trustworthy	Knows the health service
Ethical	Inspiring
Respectful	Able to receive feedback
An effective leader	Experience
Skilled in feedback	Patient
Chemistry: intellectual and emotional compatibility	
Able to challenge	
Non-judgemental	
Confidential	

Choosing your mentor

You should look for someone:

- with a track record of developing other people
- who is committed to their own personal and professional development
- who has the time and energy to fulfil their contract with you and be flexible about developing the mentoring relationship to meet your needs – not their own
- who is respected and trustworthy.

And probably:

- who has an understanding of your work or discipline, how it works and where the organisation in which you work is going
- who has up-to-date knowledge and expertise in their professional field and the NHS context.

(Adapted from Fisher H[1])

Box 2.3:   What do nurses want in a mentor?

In one study,[2] there were three vital ingredients that nurses were found to want for mentoring to be successful. If one of these was missing, the mentor relationship was said to be diminished. These ingredients are:

- attraction: admiration of the other person or a desire to emulate them in some way
- action: this includes actions taken by the mentor on behalf of the mentee, such as guiding or helping their development
- affect: the mentor has positive feelings towards the mentee and respects, encourages and supports the mentee.

Go searching for a mentor

Treat finding a mentor like searching for your perfect holiday. Do your homework. Think of all the possibilities. Is there a list of people who might be willing to be mentors that is available to you – in your organisation, in the library, on the intranet, or on a website? Decide what sort of person you need, do some research, go and visit a few people and see whether or not you think you would work well together. Try saying something like 'I am looking for a mentor – would you be willing and able to commit to this?' or 'Could I come and chat to you about the opportunities for us both if you became my mentor?' This gives you the opportunity to decide whether or not the potential mentor has the time and is willing to take on the role. But more importantly, you can find out whether or not you would be able to build a rapport with them in a mentoring relationship that would prove to be symbiotic.

Some people have more than one mentor at a time. The two mentors might be chosen for their particular characteristics or experience, or to help with very different aspects of the mentee's working life and/or career.

Should I choose someone who is like-minded?

Sometimes it is easier and more comfortable to choose somebody who has a similar personality to you or who has had similar professional or life experiences. Although it may feel easier to remain in your 'comfort zone', you may learn more from selecting a mentor who views the world differently to you and can offer a broader or more diverse perspective than your own. A mentor who challenges you will be likely to be more effective than one with whom you have a cosy relationship.

Activity 2.3: (for mentees)

What qualities will you look for in a mentor? Write them down below:

•

•

•

•

Activity 2.4: (for mentees)

Who do you know who fits these qualities? Do not limit your option to one person. He or she may already be mentoring or supervising too many people to be able to take you on or do you justice.

•

•

•

Questions you might ask a potential mentor

When you do meet up with possible mentors, base your discussion on the questions listed below or add some questions of your own to check that their views and expectations of mentoring are similar to yours. Try to find a quiet time and place to start the discussion so you have the potential mentor's full attention.

- Have you been a mentor before? (If yes) How did it go? As a result of your experience, what do you think makes mentoring work well?
- Have you had a mentor? (If yes) How did it go? As a result of your experience, what do you think makes mentoring work well?
- What jobs have your previous mentee(s) held?
- What do you think the role of a mentor is?
- How much time do you think you would be available as a mentor to me for? How often do you think we might meet and how long would we spend at a mentoring session?
- Do you feel comfortable with challenging others' views and perspectives?

The best questions will lead to a 'two-way' discussion, which gives you both a chance to match your values and perspectives and expectations.

The mentor's perspective

Being an effective mentor requires certain personal qualities and skills (*see* page 13). Whether or not you are ready to be a mentor is an important question to ask yourself before embarking on such a role. Reflect on any mentoring you have done already, and think about your own experiences of being a mentee. Ensure that you are familiar with the differences between mentoring and other management- or education-related roles – look back and reflect on Table 1.1. You need to be able to resist the temptation to give advice, and instead help the mentee to arrive at their own solutions and conclusions.

The most important thing to the mentee will be your commitment to the mentoring relationship, and so it is vital that you protect time for your mentor sessions and do not continually cancel or shorten your meetings.

The questions below may help you to decide if being a mentor is really for you.

What's in it for you as a mentor?

- Develops your own learning – by creating a two-way, co-learning relationship.
- Gives you insight into relationships.
- Satisfaction of seeing someone else 'grow'.
- An opportunity for you to be challenged in a safe environment (it is not just the mentee who can expect to be challenged).

Why would a mentee choose you?

- You have a track record for developing other people.
- You seem to be committed to others' personal and professional development.

- You seem to have the time and energy to fulfil the mentoring contract and be flexible about developing the relationship to meet the mentee's needs, not your own.
- You are well thought of and respected as trustworthy.
- You are up to date in your professional area and have a good understanding of how the NHS works.

The role of the mentor

A mentor is usually an established professional who offers a mentee opportunities to develop, stimulate and maintain their professional development through an ongoing dialogue and relationship. They will adopt all four roles described below to a varying extent, depending on the needs of the mentee.

- **An envisioner**: giving the mentee a picture of what the future can be like.
- **A standard prodder**: pushing the mentee to achieve high standards and encouraging them to take risks in order to develop.
- **A challenger**: making the mentee look more closely at their skills and the decisions they make.
- **A confidante**: good listening skills, allowing the mentee to 'open up' with any problems or concerns.

Activity 2.5: (for mentors)

What qualities do you have to enable you to be an effective mentor?

-

-

-

-

Learning points for you as a mentor

- It is not essential for mentors to have technical and/or specialist knowledge of the mentee's fields of interest or work.
- A mentor's role is to be expert at helping the mentee to learn and develop – they do not need to be in a position of seniority or authority. This role is less like 'tell him/her all you know', and more like 'help him/her to find what it is s/he needs.'
- The *quality* of the relationship is vital, more so than the background of the mentor. Learning and development is unlikely to take place without the mentee and mentor establishing mutual trust, respect and safe ethical boundaries.

The NHS perspective

A recent review of mentoring for doctors related that some organisations for which doctors work recognise the benefits of mentoring, but ask questions about the purpose, process and return on investment.[3] 'Trusts acknowledge that assessing benefits (of mentoring) to them as organisations is difficult and imprecise. Some medical managers speculate that mentoring ought to reduce negative events such as referrals to the General Medical Council, the time the medical director spends dealing with "difficult" doctors or the opportunity to air problems at an early stage, reducing the risk of major and escalating difficulties. Equally, medical and other managers acknowledge that such indicators as retention and reduced absence through illness and stress related disorders are also difficult to relate to mentoring, other factors being involved.'

Mentoring has been recommended as a general organisational approach for managing transition points in professional careers. In one study cited,[3] targeting investment in mentoring arrangements for new consultants, those working flexibly, new managers and those with performance problems were considered likely to yield considerable benefits for the costs involved.

What's in it for the mentee's line manager or employer (who is not the mentor too)?

- A mentor provides a reinforcing or alternative opinion (depends if the line manager and mentor are in touch in their daily work and whether mentoring discussions are agreed to be confidential).
- Improved relationships in the team.
- Shared responsibility in developing the mentee (line manager and mentor).
- A wider perspective of their organisation from feedback of mentor via the developing mentee.
- Enabling of transition points in employees' careers, so that performance is optimised through new roles and responsibilities being clarified and supported.

What's in it for the mentee's and/or mentor's trust (or other organisation)?

- Enhanced recruitment and retention of key staff – as those involved in mentoring feel valued and are likely to remain in the workforce. Enhanced job satisfaction for the mentors as well as the mentees.
- Reinforcement of culture change.
- Mentoring highlights a 'no blame' culture, by encouraging learning from shared experiences.
- Increased productivity of those being mentored.
- Improved communication across boundaries between disciplines or teams, etc.
- Reduced absence through illness and stress-related disorders.
- Reduction in time spent by people working across the organisation, in dealing with 'difficult' staff.

Setting up a mentoring scheme

Some organisations set up their own formal mentoring scheme, training, supporting and matching mentors and mentees, while elsewhere mentoring may be an informal arrangement between two people who have organised themselves without support or help from others.

Resources required

Creating a mentoring scheme in your trust or deanery or other organisation will require:

- expertise in understanding 'best practice' in mentoring and creating the structural components of the scheme: training, resources for protecting time and/or rewarding time spent or effort, creation of mentoring contracts, support for mentors, evaluation methods (individual and organisational)
- a range of information and support for all aspects of staff management and development (to which mentors can signpost their mentees)
- mentors: sufficient numbers of enthusiastic mentors who are prepared to apply what they have learnt about good practice in mentoring
- mentees: sufficient numbers of willing mentees who are prepared to use the opportunities arising from mentoring
- training and ongoing support programme: for mentors
- training programme: for mentees
- lead for mentoring scheme: to be responsible for organising the scheme, evaluating its achievement, assessing and rectifying problems, being a champion for obtaining/ sustaining resources and organisational commitment, linking the mentoring scheme with other organisational activities and priorities
- facilitator for mentoring scheme: project management ensuring the efficiency of the day-to-day organisation of the scheme, answering queries, recruiting and selecting mentors and mentees, organising the matching of mentor–mentee, running or commissioning training, acting as problem solver if there are mentor/ mentee/organisational issues, arranging reimbursement of expenses, reinforcing methods and techniques of good mentoring practice, etc.
- administrative support
- documentation: contracts, expense claims, templates for personal development plans or action planning.

All the people involved in the list above need adequate time to be allocated in their working lives to be able to participate and fulfil their roles and responsibilities in the mentoring scheme.

Recruiting potential mentors

The mentor needs to understand the voluntary nature of mentoring, and its developmental purpose and supportive, yet challenging nature. Different trusts and organisations require varying preparation by mentors for their role.[3] Some rely on would-be mentors' experience gained from other roles, such as academic supervision and continuing education, while others expect potential or novice mentors to participate in training and support programmes over many months. Box 2.4 lists the qualifications and experience that the majority of 16 participants in one study based in general practice[4] believed were essential or desirable for mentors of GPs at appointment.

Box 2.4: Suggested qualifications and experience for mentor of GPs at appointment[4]

1 Be working currently or within past two years as a GP
2 Have up-to-date clinical skills
3 Background in training and development
4 Have counselling skills/have been trained in counselling
5 Be well versed in general practice administration and politics
6 Have attended at least three training workshops in mentoring
7 Experience of life
8 Have self-confidence
9 Be intuitive
10 Declare not currently under investigation for any criminal offence or General Medical Council/local procedure which might bring mentoring process into disrepute

---

There is no one way to recruit mentors. Informal mentors are selected by would-be mentees, and if the mentor–mentee develop their relationship in isolation from any scheme and do not call upon any authority for resources, then there is unlikely to be any external input into the selection of such a mentor, except as informal advice from colleagues. Mentors normally volunteer, though some staff may be expected to act as mentors by some directors or organisations by virtue of their posts, such as holding developmental type roles or being academic supervisors. One report of mentoring schemes relates that 'many doctors who have put themselves forward for formal development programmes (as mentors) are self-selected. Scheme organisers ... reserve the right to recommend that doctors who have completed a course do not then become mentors if the organisers feel that they are completely out of sympathy with the principles and practice of mentorship, but this rarely happens.'[3] Another option is to integrate peer review into the training process. For example, during role play of realistic scenarios, you can include peer reports in building up a picture of the would-be mentor's suitability. Box 2.5 describes how one mentor training consultancy organises such a de-selection process after the initial training has been completed.

Box 2.5: Example of mentor recruitment and training approach by one consultancy[5]

Arcadia Alive, a human factors consultancy, is commissioned by health and other organisations to set up mentoring schemes. They recommend that recruitment and training should be a two-stage process.

1 Basic training selection
• A short application form (contact details, plus a paragraph on why the applicant wants to become a mentor, what they feel they could bring to the

continued opposite

role and what they hope to gain from the training course, and how they meet the criteria – either show evidence of the qualities listed or express willingness to learn).
- Two references asking for the referees' views on whether the would-be mentor meets the criteria.

Required criteria of potential mentors:
- good motivators, perceptive, able to support the mentoring programme objectives and fulfil the responsibilities to the mentee
- high performers, secure in their own position ... unlikely to feel threatened by, or resentful of, the mentee's opportunities
- able to establish a good and professional relationship, be sympathetic, accessible and knowledgeable about the mentee's area of interest
- good teachers, able to advise and instruct without interfering, allowing mentees to explore and pursue ideas.

2 End-of-training interview
For would be-mentors who have undertaken initial training but who have not acquired the necessary skills, or who have not demonstrated that they understand the role and responsibilities of mentoring, it will be necessary to either:
- develop an action plan with specific areas for improvement and change, and a follow-up process, or
- fail the applicant to be a mentor outright.

Training potential mentors

Some organisations recruit and train a cohort of would-be mentors before any mentees have been identified so that potential mentors learn and practise their newfound skills, then take on mentees at a later date in a formal scheme or informal way. Others prefer to teach mentorship skills to any professionals who are interested, who may then go on to co-mentor each other, each taking a turn to be mentor or mentee in a mentoring session. Others recruit mentors just ahead of the mentees so that the 'live' mentoring enhances their learning within the mentoring scheme.[3]

An outline of a typical initial training programme for mentors is given in Chapter 7 (*see* page 145).[5] The purpose of the day is for potential mentors to understand the meaning of mentoring (as described in Chapter 1), develop a positive attitude to mentoring and learn the skills to be an effective mentor (*see* Chapters 3 and 4). Mentoring schemes differ in length of training and the amount of time they provide to practise mentor skills, and the emphasis they place on organisational development. Some of the variation can be accounted for by the nature and background of the trainer as well as the commissioning body, and the extent of life experience of those selected to be mentors. Some courses are run in house, others engage outside consultants as trainers or sponsor staff to attend external courses. Many continue with opportunities for refreshment and practise of skills, and peer support sessions to share successes and problems and review progress – within limits of preserving confidentiality between mentor and mentee. Some trusts prefer to commission a visiting consultant or their organisation to establish and support the mentoring scheme administration and development.[3]

If your mentoring scheme adopts the job description of a mentor we recommend in Chapter 7 (*see* page 139), then there could be an opportunity in the initial training to assess the would-be mentor's knowledge and skills against the competencies described. The facilitator might work with the mentor to agree what further professional development the mentor might need to uprate their competency as a mentor and how they will address knowledge and skill gaps. You can read more about this in Chapters 3 and 4, where we consider what tools and techniques might enable you to perform effectively as a mentor.

Training mentees

The terms 'mentoring' and 'mentor' are used in many different ways, and potential mentors and mentees may misunderstand the meaning of a mentoring relationship, what their commitment will be and lack the knowledge and skills to make mentoring work. So it is just as important to train potential mentees as it is to train the potential or novice mentors.

An outline of a typical initial training session run over a half-day is given in Chapter 7 on page 149. The purpose of the day is for the mentees to understand the meaning of mentoring (as described in Chapter 1), develop a positive attitude to mentoring, evolve reasonable expectations of mentoring expecting a developmental and challenging relationship, and learn the skills to be an effective mentee (*see* Chapter 6).

Matching mentors and mentees

A recent overview of mentoring schemes reports that 'techniques for bringing mentors and mentees together formally vary considerably. They range from encouraging mentees to exercise free choice from a pool of potential mentors all the way to allocation of the next available mentor from the top of a list. All schemes claim to allow both participants to decline the other ... Some schemes require an initial meeting and then a decision is taken whether to continue. In the co-mentoring arrangements, participants get to know each other during the development course and then form co-mentoring dyads or triads ... Scheme organisers and administrators often exercise judgement about who will suit whom. Ease of meeting is important to the success of a mentoring relationship, so you need to consider such factors as:

- geographical proximity
- transportation
- flexible/shift working
- commitments outside work.'[3]

Some mentoring schemes are specialty-specific with both mentors and mentees from the same discipline, but other schemes deliberately avoid this. The Royal College of Obstetricians and Gynaecologists has set up a mentoring service for doctors in difficulty, as described in Box 2.6.

Box 2.6: The Royal College of Obstetricians and Gynaecologists (RCOG) mentoring scheme[6]

The RCOG is proactive in seeking out fellows and members of the College who are in difficulty and who may need help and support. Doctors may self-refer, or be referred by their trust or healthcare organisation, or the College may become aware of their difficulty from national or local press or the General Medical Council website.

   The College writes to the doctor in difficulty and invites him/her to volunteer to be linked to a mentor. A mentor is proposed who appears to match the would-be mentee's needs and timeframe. The mentee makes the first contact with the mentor. The initial cohort of 23 mentors attended a four-day intensive training course to launch the UK-wide scheme.

'Many hospital trust-based schemes offer mentors only from the same trust, though this may be from another site some distance away. Seniors taking on new management roles may be offered a mentor outside the employing organisation ... It appears to be important to have a wide selection of mentors, but matching for the same gender and same ethnic origin does not seem to be important or often requested.'[3]

   You need to take mentor–mentee preferences into account as far as possible within the limits of who is available, but further research is needed to realise the extent to which the nature of mentor–mentee matching affects the achievements and outcomes of mentoring from individual mentee, mentor and organisational perspectives.

Confirming the joining arrangements

After the recruitment, selection and training processes, whoever is organising the mentoring scheme will want to confirm the arrangements with the mentors and mentees. You may use the documentation included in Chapter 7 to agree terms and conditions, and the resources that relate to the individual mentor or mentee concerned – *see* page 77 for the sort of resources that need to be available.

   Using a tool such as the log record sheet (*see* page 154) for example, is a simple way to confirm arrangements such as dates, times, venues and duration of mentoring sessions. If *you* have to change, cancel or shorten any of these meetings you have a clear record of how often that is happening. If it becomes apparent that *your mentor* is changing, cancelling or shortening your sessions then you need to discuss their commitment to the process. No matter how skilful a mentor is, if he or she is unable to give you the time you need, then the potential benefits of the mentoring relationship will be significantly reduced.

   When confirming the arrangements you will need to give careful consideration to how often you meet. It may be that you will benefit from meeting someone who you believe to be a skilled mentor who can only commit to a session every 12 weeks, rather than meeting another possible mentor who might suit you less well every six weeks.

   The items in the job description of a mentor (*see* Chapter 7, page 139) may be included in the mentor's current job description within the employing organisation or be issued as a stand-alone job description for the mentor post, however part-time it is. The mentor should be issued with a brief contract by those organising the scheme, describing the terms of the position, code of confidentiality, time allocation (*see* page 151 for an example).

The mentee should be issued with a letter of confirmation from the scheme organiser so that he or she knows the limits of the scheme and what the mentee's rights are.

Making mentoring sessions work

Ground rules that mentor and mentee should discuss before they start

Start by agreeing ground rules for meeting and how or whether you will record your meeting. Clarify the objectives and outcomes that you both want to cover. You may wish to revisit the ground rules from time to time, or at the start of each session, to check that you both continue to be happy with your agreement. The ground rules should cover:

- main purpose and focus of the meetings
- expectations of mentor and mentee
- commitment of mentor and mentee to the mentoring process
- confidentiality and any exceptions – in both a personal and professional capacity (*see* page 150)
- how to exit or opt out
- who has responsibility for arranging meetings
- frequency of meetings
- length of meetings (e.g. 60–120 minutes)
- location of meetings
- arrangements for cancellations (either mentor or mentee)
- number of cancellations before the mentoring contract is reviewed
- documentation/record keeping – what records and who is keeping them
- how to evaluate the mentoring relationship by feedback from mentor or mentee
- what records or feedback will be passed to the scheme organiser (if there is one, for accountability purposes, especially if the mentor is employed or mentoring is happening in work time)
- length of time the mentoring contract will span
- personal boundaries
- any potential conflicts of interest and agree action (*see* text below).

Confidentiality is a tricky issue. On the one hand the mentor and mentee need to develop a trusting relationship where confidences are welcomed and respected. On the other hand, if patient safety is threatened from the mentee's clinical practice, and that risk persists, a health professional has an ethical obligation to take action to remove that risk to patient safety and may break confidentiality if there is no other way forward. This conflict and any other emanating from the mentor's and mentee's roles need to be discussed and the limits of confidentiality agreed as relevant. The limits of confidentiality are considered in more detail on page 92.

Activity 2.6: (for mentor or mentee)

What ground rules are essential for you? Have a go at writing them down drawing from the list above.

-

-

-

-

-

-

-

-

Preparing for the mentoring session as a mentor

It is important that as a mentor you are as prepared for each meeting as the mentee. Although it is primarily the mentee's responsibility to set out an agenda, he or she will probably be relying on you as the mentor to guide the meeting. Figure 2.1 may help to provide some structure to help move the meeting forward. Providing a relaxed atmosphere is crucial, but equally it is important not to spend too much time chitchatting before you move on to the purpose of the meeting.

Remember that the issues are to be explored from the mentee's perspective. Do not try and put yourself in their shoes and make assumptions about how they feel. Keep clarifying what is being said so that you both obtain a full picture.

At the end of the meeting it is important that the actions are agreed by both of you. The mentor should not go away with more actions than the mentee. As far as possible,

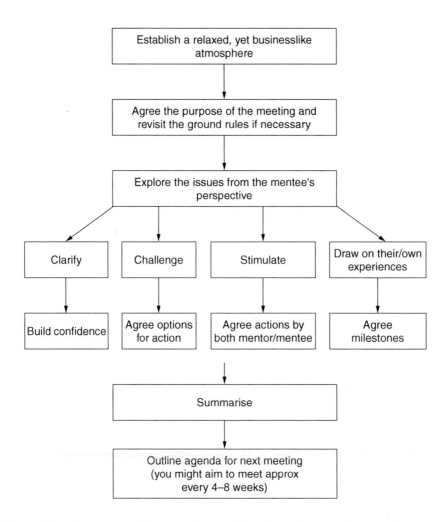

Figure 2.1:   The process of the mentoring meeting – from the mentor's perspective.

all actions are the mentee's responsibility. In the long term, you are not being helpful by saying 'let me do that for you'. Do not take on the role of the parent. Encouraging the mentee to take responsibility for themselves and their own learning is a key element to effective mentoring.

Preparing for the mentoring session as a mentee

A common framework used for mentoring follows three stages:

1   **exploration**: when the mentor listens, and prompts the mentee with questions
2   **new understanding**: when the mentor listens and challenges the mentee, recognises strengths and weaknesses of the ideas, shares experiences, establishes priorities, identifies development needs, and gives information and supportive feedback

3 **action planning**: when the mentor encourages new ways of thinking, helps the
   mentee reach a solution, agrees goals and decides action plans.

As a mentee, you will need to make the most of the precious time spent with your mentor.
Good preparation will enable you to participate fully in all three stages. Box 2.7
summarises a good example of a mentoring model, devised by Parsloe and Wray.[7]

Areas that a mentee may wish to discuss

- Work-related issues.
- Career development.
- Time management.
- Leadership styles.
- Learning styles.
- Issues arising from the mentoring discussions, for example:
  - feedback from patients or colleagues or mentor
  - outcomes of patient story telling and observation of care/practice.
- Shadowing experiences.
- Political issues.
  - understanding the politics of the organisation
  - the translation of national policies to a local level.
- Networking opportunities.

Parsloe and Wray model of mentoring[7]

The Parsloe and Wray model of mentoring is a user-friendly approach. It provides
some overall guidance to ensure that the mentoring process completes a full cycle.
It is a common error to concentrate on one aspect of the issues, whether it is the
problem, the plan, or the past. This model ensures that the mentee and mentor see a
problem or issue in perspective and work through it to the end. If an end is not
achievable then the model will aid the evaluation of the process as far as they can get,
and assess what has been achieved.

   Many models used in mentoring have their roots in psychology, generally attempt-
ing to challenge negative thoughts or self-limiting beliefs in the pursuit of fulfilling the
potential of the mentee. The Parsloe and Wray model has been widely used with senior
executives to help improve their personal performance, and likewise the performance
of their organisation.

Box 2.7:   The Parsloe and Wray mentoring model[7]

Stages   *Organisational and qualification mentoring*
Stage 1   Gain understanding and acceptance. Confirm the personal develop-
             ment plan (PDP) and establish what are the short-term and longer-
             term aims of the PDP
Stage 2   Motivate for action. Encourage self-management of learning
Stage 3   Support the plan. Provide support throughout your mentoring contract
Stage 4   Review and maintain momentum. Assist in the evaluation of outcomes
             of mentoring

Stage 1: Establish the aims of mentoring

- The mentor may be involved at any stage during preparation – but the primary role at this stage is simply to help the mentee to establish their longer-term developmental aims.
- The mentor should prepare for their role by anticipating and identifying the likely needs of the mentee. This will include helping the mentee to develop a self-awareness and acceptance of their existing strengths and weaknesses.
- The mentor will encourage the development of self-awareness and responsibility in the mentee by using honest, open questioning and feedback.
- The mentor should keep their mentee on track with their personal development plan (PDP) by encouraging them to formulate goals that are SMART (Specific, Measurable, Achievable, Relevant and Timescaled). It may be that setting goals needs to be taken one step at a time, reflecting on the process of goal setting, likely barriers and ways of overcoming those barriers.
- Establish the boundaries between the mentor's role and that of other professionals (look back at Table 1.1), with the mentor signposting the mentee to a range of information and support agencies that are available, as necessary.

Activity 2.7: (for mentees)

Make a note of your aims at the start of mentoring. It will be a useful portrait of your learning curve to refer back to, while you are in this mentoring relationship.

-

-

-

Stage 2: Encourage the mentee's self-management or self-direction of learning and motivate action

- A good mentor–mentee relationship is characterised by the extent to which it allows the mentee to self-manage the process. The mentor can ask probing questions that encourage the mentee to think ahead, anticipate and plan aspects of getting maximum benefit and action from their PDP or any learning activities in which they are engaged.

- The mentor should ensure that mentoring activities do not compromise the boundaries between a mentee and their line/senior manager. Mentees should always be encouraged to work out their own solutions to problems with line managers or other colleagues as appropriate.
- Both mentor and mentee should remember that a mentor is a 'sounding board' – not a trouble-shooter.
- Mentoring conversations should be undertaken in confidence so that genuine trust can exist (but *see* ground rules on pages 24 and 92 for limits to confidentiality in the health service). Adopting a genuinely objective, confidential, impartial role may not always be easy in practice, but it is essential. A clear contract which defines boundaries and expectations of both mentor and mentee is essential from the outset.

Stage 3: Provide ongoing support

- The mentor needs to be available to provide support during the mentoring relationship. In practice, this means agreeing to a schedule of meetings that are mutually convenient. You may agree that email, instant messaging or telephone contact is acceptable within agreed parameters.
- The timing, pace and level of support/information offered is critical.
- The mentor will need to be sensitive to the culture, beliefs, capabilities, aspirations and learning preferences of the mentee in order to match their learning style (*see* page 120). The mentor must guard against imposing their preferred methods or preferences of learning on the mentee. A mentor with a *theorist* learning style could mistakenly recommend research or reading to a mentee who prefers to be an *activist* learner. Ideally, mentors should be knowledgeable about learning styles and sufficiently self-aware to be able to adapt to the learning style of their mentee.
- Mentors will sometimes be asked by the mentee to provide advice and guidance. The key here is for the mentor to provide such guidance only when asked and not to impose it on the mentee in a mistaken attempt to appear knowledgeable or helpful.
- The mentor must take care not to provide such an extent of support that the mentee comes to feel *dependent* on the mentor.
- Agree methods of contact to deal with urgent or unforeseen difficulties that are appropriate to debate within the mentoring contract.
- A key role for the mentor is helping the mentee to deal with mistakes and setbacks. The mentoring relationship should be 'non-judgemental' and 'risk-free', thereby allowing the mentee to treat mistakes and setbacks as real opportunities to learn.
- A mentor should try to build self-confidence and motivation in the mentee at all times. This is essential to helping the mentee to assume a positive attitude which will provide a basis for future learning and development.

Stage 4: Assist in evaluating outcomes of mentoring, reviewing and maintaining momentum

- The mentor should encourage the mentee to reflect on their learning and progress. The use of reflective questions or reflective diaries can help mentees to analyse any barriers that crop up.
- The mentor should remind the mentee of the value of self/peer assessment of their standards of performance. Encourage them to try out 360 degree feedback (*see* page 87).
- The mentor should help the mentee to quantify the benefits of their learning or development for themselves *and* their organisation.
- The mentoring relationship may come to an end at the completion of the mentoring contract or with a job change, etc. A skilled mentor can turn an ending into a celebration of success and a recognition of the mutual benefits (to the mentee and their employing organisation) gained through the relationship. The mentor can also encourage the mentee to set new challenges and career goals for the future.
- The mentor should encourage the mentee to set outcomes for what they hope to achieve from the mentoring relationship at their initial meeting. Discuss how appropriate and realistic the outcomes envisaged are at that meeting and in later ones as relevant.
- The mentor should help the mentee prepare to evaluate the mentoring relationship and overall benefits of mentoring to the individual – *see* Box 2.8 for ideas to aid evaluation and analysis at the completion of the mentoring sessions. A mentee might respond to the questions in Box 2.8 and then seek views from their mentor or other colleagues who know them well.

Box 2.8:   A structure for the final evaluation of the mentoring sessions

- What did you actually do in the mentoring sessions?
- What had you hoped to achieve from this mentoring relationship?
- What did you actually achieve?
- Were there any unexpected learning points?
- What changes have you made as a result of your mentoring sessions?
- How would you describe the personal benefits?
- How would you describe the organisational benefits from you being mentored?
- What do you think you could do next to build on your achievements?
- Have you any outstanding plans that you have not yet put into place? What has stopped your plans from happening?

The role of the mentor using a behavioural matrix

The behavioural matrix in Figure 2.2 is based on the qualities required of a mentor.[8] The mentor will probably work their way around the whole matrix at various stages of the relationship. Where they lie in the matrix will be determined by the needs of the mentee, but if the mentor believes they are operating predominantly within the active roles then it is important that they take a step back and reassess their relationship and roles. It is vital to encourage the mentee to take on more responsibility and ownership

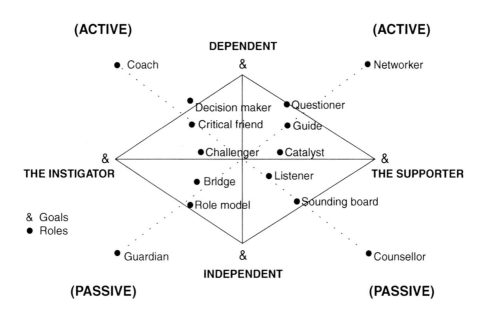

Figure 2.2: The role of the mentor presented as a behavioural matrix[8] (adapted from Clutterbuck 2000).

of the meetings and in meeting the outcomes. One of the fundamental outcomes of any mentoring relationship is for the mentee to develop and grow, therefore they are there to learn and not receive teaching. To gain full benefit from the relationship, the mentee needs to be ready, willing and able to work with a mentor. As the relationship develops, the mentor should be assuming more *passive* roles such as 'listener', 'guardian' and 'sounding board'.

One of the most important aspects of a mentor's role is to help the mentee become as independent as possible. Initially the mentor may give a lot of guidance and have to ask most of the questions ('questioner'), but the aim is to lessen this type of input as the mentee's confidence increases. Some techniques the mentor can use to ensure they are not always playing the *active* roles include:

- encouraging mentees to make decisions and find answers for themselves
- turning the mentee's questions back to the mentee, e.g. 'What do you think? What would you do?'
- encouraging the mentee to keep a reflective diary, thinking how and where in the matrix of Figure 2.2 they best learn and where they are making progress. This will help to build their confidence and self-reliance
- increasing the length of time between meetings as the mentee becomes more confident, which can enable the mentee to take on the more active roles.

Activity 2.8: (for mentors)

Figure 2.2 reflects the variety of active and passive roles within the mentor's scope. The aim is for the mentor to work through the diamond-shaped matrix in the figure. The mentor should start out as the *instigator* at the beginning of the mentoring relationship and work through to become the *supporter* in an established relationship. The mentee will be likely to be *dependent* in a new relationship and will progress to being *independent*, helped by the skill of the mentor, working through the roles within the diamond-shaped matrix, after which the mentor can adopt more passive roles. Other peripheral roles outside mentoring lie outside the diamond shape. Think where you lie in the behavioural matrix of Figure 2.2.

- Are you displaying more active or passive roles in your mentor sessions?

- Are you achieving your goal in becoming the *supporter* rather than the *instigator?*

- Is your mentee working towards independence?

Recognising common problems in relation to mentoring

In one mentoring initiative,[9] there were a number of common matters that prevented people from becoming involved. These were:

- 'pressure of work' reported by one would-be mentee; pace of work and non-availability of time
- not the culture in many professions
- lack of access to informal networks
- threat of would-be mentee being seen as 'in need', exposing vulnerability
- opportunity for mentoring never cropped up
- threat of being in competition with people for jobs or posts, who may have been your mentor or mentee in the past
- mentoring being seen as something offered to junior people
- terminology off-putting
- personal risk – fear of mentee in relation to lapse of confidentiality
- not knowing who to go to or how to arrange to have a mentor.

Other pitfalls in mentoring include:

- poor planning and preparation
- poor selection of mentors and mentees
- limited clarity of roles
- too little or too much formality
- failure to set and measure clear outcomes.

Common pitfalls in mentoring relationships

- Failure to establish rapport.
- Under- or over-management.
- Poor objective setting.
- Lack of time.
- Breach of confidentiality.
- Line manager feeling excluded or threatened.

Overcoming possible problems arising in a mentor–mentee relationship

Below are suggestions to help you overcome some of the problems or issues that might crop up at any time throughout your mentoring contract.[10] You may have other solutions or need to address problems that do not appear below.

- Time commitment ... so assess the time needed realistically and plan for it.
- Conflict of interests if mentor is 'line manager' of mentee ... so clarify your relationship. If it is impossible to establish sufficient trust, then you need to find a different mentor/mentee match.
- Strained relationship between mentor and mentee ... so agree boundaries to develop the right balance between empathy and intimacy.
- The 'halo' effect ... both mentor and mentee should be aware that the mentee may attribute a 'halo' to the mentor, whose opinions may be seen as absolute answers. Discuss and defuse this tendency.
- Other colleagues being jealous of close relationship of mentor–mentee ... beware that the mentee is not seen by his or her colleagues as getting an unfair amount of attention and support and try not to let your mentor–mentee relationship fuel resentment.
- Criticism of mentee by mentor ... both should be aware of the sensitivities of the mentee to any criticism and take the utmost care with formal and informal, verbal and non-verbal feedback. Discuss problems analytically without bringing personalities into it. Use a constructive feedback technique (*see* page 53).
- Undue sexual attraction ... take care to act professionally at all times.
- Dislike by one or each of the other ... liking each other is essential. Discontinue a mentor–mentee relationship where any sort of dislike creeps in.

Reviewing your mentoring relationship – is it working?

You might carry out an informal review together every 3–6 months. Think about your last session.

- How did the last session begin?
- What did the mentee bring to the session in the form of preparation?
- Did the session follow the mentee's agenda?
- Were any deviations from the mentee's agenda acknowledged and negotiated?

- What was the balance between listening, support, information and challenge in your (the mentor) responses?
- Did you think this balance was appropriate in the relationship and the needs of the mentee?
- What specific interventions did you use, as the mentor?

Activity 2.9: (for mentors or mentees)

Is your mentoring relationship working? Mentor and/or mentee should give their views of themselves in the mentor–mentee relationship, then feed back to each other. You might do this at intervals throughout your relationship.

- What are the strengths of your relationship?

- What areas need to be developed?

Evaluating a mentoring scheme

The previous section and Box 2.8 and accompanying text gave some ideas for evaluation of a particular mentoring relationship. You might plan an evaluation in a wider way by generalising from the four levels described by Kirkpatrick in the hierarchial model (Figure 2.3). Kirkpatrick described four levels of evaluation in which the complexity of the behavioural change increases as the evaluation strategies used ascend to a higher level.[11] Evaluation of reaction will include satisfaction or happiness with the mentoring process or relationships; evaluation of learning will cover knowledge or skills acquired by mentees and mentors. Evaluation of behaviour will include the transfer of learning to the workplace; while evaluation of results will cover the transfer or impact of the activity on improvements in patient care or society.[10,11]

Using this model, you might evaluate the structural components of the mentoring scheme – the processes, recruitment and selection of mentors and mentees, training of mentors and mentees, support systems, monitoring of processes in Level 1-type evaluation measures.

You might evaluate the extent of knowledge and skills, personal and professional development gained by mentees, mentors and others in the organisation as a result of the mentoring process in Level 2-type evaluation measures. This might include monitoring the performance of mentors, and the extent to which they apply their knowledge and skills in their relationships with mentees.

You might evaluate the extent to which learning and development is transferred to their workplaces and what changes and improvements are made and sustained by Level 3-type evaluation measures.

You might evaluate tangible improvements to patient care and society in Level-4 type evaluation measures. As you go 'up' the hierarchy, evaluation becomes more difficult, as it is rarely possible to attribute gains and achievements solely to one factor such as mentoring, when there are many other developmental opportunities, support, changes and pressures in play which have little to do with any mentoring process.

You will probably fix the levels of evaluation you aim for according to the purpose of the mentoring process with which you are involved. If you are a mentor–mentee pair with an informal arrangement outside any formal scheme, you might organise Level 1 or 2-type evaluation measures. Whereas if you are responsible for establishing an organisation-wide scheme, you should endeavour to set up evaluation at all four levels, by gathering information for structural, personal and organisational markers of performance from a wide variety of sources.

Although it is difficult to do in a meaningful way without disproportionate effort to the mentoring process itself, evaluation is essential if you are to be able to review the success of the scheme, improve its operation and make a case for its continuation.

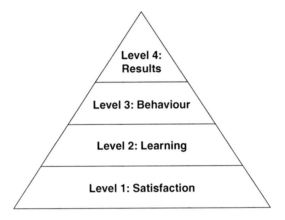

Figure 2.3:   Kirkpatrick's hierarchy of levels of evaluation[11]

Encouraging the success of the mentoring scheme

There are a number of factors that can possibly influence the success of a mentoring scheme. These include:

- a thorough needs assessment, to establish whether the organisation as a whole feels that mentoring is an appropriate response to their needs
- publicity for the existence of the mentoring scheme and the positive benefits, both initially and on an ongoing basis
- a professional standard of mentoring: thorough basic training, plus ongoing supervision and support, and regular appraisal of mentors
- monitoring, evaluation and quality control of the service, ideally with feedback from mentees as an integral component in improving the mentoring scheme and sustaining standards.

References

1 Fisher H (2002) Birmingham City Council. Unpublished.

2 Darling AL (1984) What do nurses want in a mentor? *J Nurs Admin.* **October**: 42–4.

3 Oxley J, Fleming B, Golding L *et al.* (2003) *Mentoring for Doctors: enhancing the benefit.* Improving Working Lives for Doctors. Doctors' Forum, Department of Health, London.

4 Chambers R, Tavabie A, See S and Hughes S (2004) Template for a competency based job description for mentors of GPs using the NHS Knowledge and Skills Framework. *Education for Primary Care.* **15**: 220–30.

5 Schwartz & Brisby/Arcadia Alive Ltd, Arcadia Alive, Human Factors Consultancy, Parkfield Centre, Park Street, Stafford ST17 4AL.

6 Bowen-Simpkins P, Mellows H and Dhillon C (2004) Royal College of Obstetricians and Gynaecologists mentoring scheme. *BMJ Careers.* S56.

7 Parsloe E and Wray W (2000) *Coaching and Mentoring – practical methods to improve learning.* Kogan Page, London.

8 Clutterbuck D (2002) A Guide to Mentoring. Learning from Experience – mentoring for change in the new NHS. National Mentoring Conference presentation, London. Unpublished.

9 Matthews F, Evans L and Garside M (1993) *A Project to Develop Guidance on Mentoring for Senior Executives.* Yorkshire Regional Health Authority, Leeds.

10 Mohanna K, Wall D and Chambers R (2003) *Teaching Made Easy. A Manual for Health Professionals* (2e). Radcliffe Medical Press, Oxford.

11 Kirkpatrick DJ (1967) Evaluation of training. In: R Craig and J Bittel (eds) *Training and Development Handbook.* McGraw-Hill, New York.

3

Developing your competence as a mentor with good communication and development skills

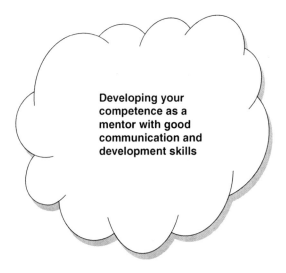

Developing your
competence as a
mentor with good
communication and
development skills

Setting out your knowledge and skills as a mentor in the context of the NHS

The emphasis is on the mentor helping the mentee to develop their own thinking and find their own way. Being a mentor is not about teaching the mentee new skills or acting as a patron to ease the mentee's career path by special favours. So, the knowledge and skills you need to develop and maintain as a mentor should be enhanced by your willingness to promote the mentee's self-directed learning and development and to share your values and beliefs, as in Box 3.1.

Box 3.1:   Remember that mentoring is:

The process by which an experienced, highly regarded, empathic person (the mentor) guides another individual (the mentee) in the development and re-examination of their own ideas, learning, and personal and professional development. The mentor, who often but not necessarily, works in the same organisation or field as the mentee, achieves this by listening and talking in confidence to the mentee.[1]

The mentor and mentee need to be clear about their respective roles and responsibilities before drawing up the contract or setting off together. Once you know what is expected of you as a mentor you can consider whether you already have the right knowledge and skills or need some updating or training.

As a mentor, you might be acting in a voluntary or a paid capacity. The time spent on mentoring might be an integral part of your day job as a manager or educationalist. Whatever your circumstances, there will be someone with whom you agree your role and responsibilities, probably whoever is employing you in your day job or as a mentor, but you will at least agree the scope of your role with your mentee.

Linking the competencies of a mentor to the NHS Knowledge and Skills Framework

A tool you might use to describe the knowledge and skills you will need for your role and responsibilities as a mentor is the NHS Knowledge and Skills Framework (KSF).[2] This framework seems to be an appropriate tool for describing the characteristics of any employed post in the NHS and is part of the NHS Agenda for Change initiative.[3] Under Agenda for Change, staff employed by the NHS (excluding doctors, independent contractors and their staff) will be placed in one of eight pay bands, depending on their knowledge, responsibility, skills and effort needed for their job. The KSF is intended to be used as part of a structured approach to training, development and review, with the overall aim of improving the consistency and quality of services to patients. Although the six core dimensions and other specific dimensions of the KSF are based on what knowledge and skills staff are currently expected to possess, adopting the KSF will have significant implications for revealing previously unfilled and/or unrecognised training needs in relation to all health professionals, managers and the non-professional workforce.

The KSF can be utilised to describe a competent mentor in the NHS, whatever the setting or professional group, or seniority of the mentor–mentee relationship. A literature search of the descriptions of a competent mentor in the context of doctors found that using the tool broadened the range of knowledge and skills expected of a mentor of general practitioners from others' descriptions. The result of this study was that all six core dimensions of the KSF and three of the other specific dimensions were found to be relevant to the job description of a mentor – as shown in Box 3.2.[4]

Each dimension of the KSF is further described in levels. Each level starts by describing Level 1 and shows successively more advanced levels of knowledge and skills and/or increasing complexity of application of knowledge and skills to the demands of work. The content of each level builds on that of the preceding level. The number of levels in each of the 22 dimensions of the sixth version of the KSF varies between four and five.[2] (The seventh version of the KSF has 31 dimensions.)

The description of your role and responsibilities based on the KSF will allow performance management of you as a mentor, as well as facilitating your professional development, as you identify learning needs by comparing your current knowledge and skills against those expected now and in the near future. You might keep a portfolio of your learning and work as a mentor, showing how you meet the defined levels of knowledge and skills in your job description. You could include a section in your main job description of your roles and responsibilities as a mentor based on the KSF. This should then map easily into your main job description if it, too, is based on the KSF. If you are employed by the NHS, this approach should enable you to clarify with your employer how you are operating as a mentor over and above your everyday job. See page 139 for an example job description and person specification, based on the NHS KSF.

Box 3.2: Descriptions of knowledge and skills of a mentor, organised under the NHS Knowledge and Skills Framework (KSF)[4]

The first six are core dimensions, and are followed by three specific dimensions.

1 Communication: consistently practise good communication skills with mentees and your organisation (Level 4)
2 Personal and people development: develop own and others' knowledge and practice across professional and organisational boundaries in relation to mentoring (Level 5)
3 Health, safety and security: promote others' health, safety and security in relation to mentoring, through risk management (Level 1)
4 Service development: develop and improve NHS services through mentoring (Level 3)
5 Quality improvement: demonstrate personal commitment to quality improvement, offering others advice and support as integral part of mentoring (Level 4)
6 Equality, diversity and rights: enable others to exercise their rights, and promote equal opportunities and diversity through mentoring (Level 3)
7 Promotion of self-care and peer support: encourage others to promote their own current and future health and wellbeing through mentoring (Level 1)
8 Partnership and support: develop and sustain partnership working with mentees and their organisation (e.g. trust, deanery) (Level 1)
9 Leadership skills: lead others in the development of knowledge, ideas and work practice as integral part of mentoring (Level 2)

Although you might demonstrate that you are competent as a mentor by referring to evidence of your knowledge and skills matched against the list of competencies in Box 3.2, that does not ensure that you will perform consistently well. One of the downsides of tools and frameworks such as the NHS KSF is that they imply that performance can be anticipated and measured, whereas in reality in healthcare it is difficult to do so in a complex and changing health setting.

Being competent and performing well as a mentor

Being competent is the 'ability to perform the tasks and roles required to the expected standard',[5] where knowledge and skills are components of competence. Performing consistently well will depend on your personal application and morale as a mentor, the availability of resources and support such as training and protected time, and the expectations and preparedness of your mentee. We know that it is not sufficient to have knowledge and know-how (competence), but that we also need to apply our knowledge and skills in practice as consistently good performance in action. As a mentor you need to possess high-order professional judgement as well as the core competencies to be *able to apply* your knowledge and skills consistently in appropriate ways with a range of mentees. As a mentor, you will have many attributes over and above those described in Box 3.2 relating to the KSF, and be competent to deal with complex situations that may crop up between you and the mentee, and consider the mentee's personal experiences.

Having self-confidence and being intuitive were rated as being essential or desirable attributes by all but one of the respondents to the study cited earlier.[4] Being a mentor does not mean being significantly older than the mentee with lots of years of experience. Although the study found that most of the respondents thought it was desirable for a mentor to have experience of life, none thought it essential and some thought it irrelevant. The literature seems to be divided on the issue. Many authors have described a mentor–mentee relationship as a mentor–novice or mentor–protégé relationship, while others have emphasised the facilitatory professional relationship between mentor and mentee.[4,6-8]

We have set out the tools and techniques that will be useful to you as a mentor for developing your knowledge and skills, under the nine headings of the relevant dimensions of the NHS KSF (*see* Box 3.2). You should read through our descriptions of what each dimension of knowledge and skills might entail. Then consider how your own knowledge and skills match up. If you have a learning need, we offer several alternative tools and techniques that you might build your knowledge and skills or positive attitude on, for that specific dimension.

Dimension 1: Communication: consistently practise good communication skills (Level 4)[2,4]

Effective communication skills

Consistently practise effective communication skills with your mentee by:

- understanding and applying good interpersonal communication: recognising and taking account of the mentee's favoured interpersonal style in order to optimise communication between you both. Summarising what the mentee says to check that you are both on the same wavelength
- using supportive, non-verbal body language
- using active listening
- establishing rapport with your mentee
- giving constructive feedback
- recognising and managing areas of resistance and conflict within the discussion process sensitively
- challenging the mentee's beliefs and plans constructively.[4]

Consider the extent to which you:

- have the knowledge and skills
- practise them – in your relationship with your mentee and in your everyday working life in other aspects of your job (you might substitute 'colleague' or 'member of staff' for 'mentee' in the list above).

Complete your audit checklist below in Table 3.1.

How expert are you? Think how expert you are for each aspect of effective communication listed in the left-hand column of Table 3.1.

- Aware? If you are merely 'aware' you might be aware that the particular knowledge and/or skill is important and have undertaken some preliminary reading and learning, but are not yet confident, practised or skilled in employing that feature of effective communication.
- Competent? If you are 'competent' you will have a good basic knowledge and be skilled in communicating with a typical mentee.
- Expert? If you are an 'expert' you will have an enormous range of experience and intuitive grasp of situations. You will be able to interpret and synthesise information and handle a wide range of communication problems in different contexts.[9]

How frequently do you use that aspect of effective communication? Think how often you employ that feature of effective communication with others at work. Think more widely than mentoring, and of your interactions with colleagues of all levels of seniority and patients. Is it at least daily or at least weekly or at least monthly? The more such knowledge and skills are part of your normal behaviour, the more likely they will feature naturally and consistently in your mentoring relationship when you meet up with your mentee(s).

Make your assessment more objective: seek others' views of your competence or performance in relation to effective communication. You might simply ask someone else who knows you well to complete a second copy of the audit Table 3.1 and compare your pre-completed table with their perspective of you – and, of course, discuss any differences with them so that you can learn from their input. You might seek feedback from your mentee towards the end of your mentoring relationship, or from others for whom you have a role or responsibility, such as in line management, educational supervision, appraisal or coaching.

Table 3.1: Self-check of own knowledge and skills in respect of communication between you as mentor and your mentee(s)

Aspect of communication	How expert are you? Aware? Competent? Expert?	How frequently do you use these? At least every day? Weekly? Monthly?
Understand and apply good interpersonal communication		
Use active listening		
Establish rapport with mentee		
Use non-verbal body language		
Give constructive feedback		
Recognise and manage conflict		
Challenge mentee's beliefs constructively		

General tips for improving your communication skills[10]

We all think we know about communication skills – and are often baffled when some-one misinterprets something we have said or done. No one should be complacent and think they cannot improve their communication skills. You can grade people into being at one of three levels.[11]

1   Unskilled. People at this level use whatever methods come naturally – good or bad. They have little or no insight into the effect that their communication has on other people. They tend to blame others for failures or dismiss others as hopeless or incapable of changing.
2   Using acquired tricks. At this level people have learnt some useful communication skills, but they tend to apply them uncritically without observing the effect or noting feedback from others.
3   The skilful communicator has a wide range of appropriate behaviours that can be tailored to the situation and modified according to the feedback received. It may sometimes be correct to give didactic orders (e.g. to shout 'fire – everyone out') or to drop gentle hints to someone where there is a sensitive issue.

You can learn how to observe, evaluate and change how you communicate with other people. Receiving feedback from others helps to make the necessary changes. Knowing about the signs that indicate someone's background mental state can help you to understand not just what is said, but the feelings behind the words. Consider the verbal and non-verbal aspects of communication, as described in Figure 3.1.

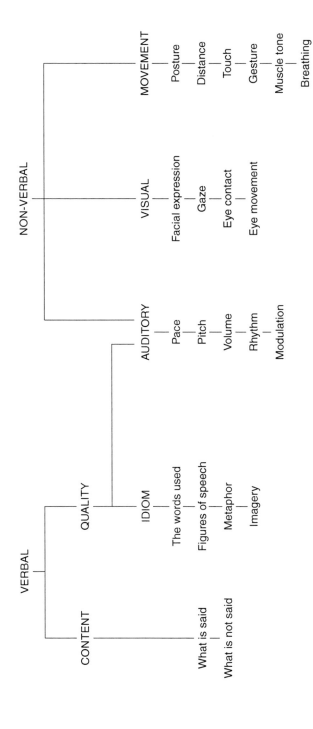

Note: bear in mind that cultural factors may influence what is happening (e.g. the amount of eye contact, gesture or touch may be altered according to the culture of origin or adoption).

Figure 3.1:   Signs of the mental state in communication.

The meaning of language[10]

Most of the time we understand what people say, but sometimes our 'wires get crossed'.[12] Some examples of poor language skills are as follows.

*   **Taking things literally**. The answer to 'Have you seen that file I put down?' is not 'Yes', but 'It's over there on the table'.
*   **Action meanings**. People often use action statements when they do not like to ask for things directly. Saying 'It's very fresh in here with the window open' can be a request for the window to be shut, and the speaker will be quite offended if you reply 'Yes, it's nice to have fresh air coming in'.
*   **Connotative meanings**. These can suggest emotions but express what is said and what is meant differently. People who use metaphors implying that the work-place is a war zone (e.g. we will attack this problem on several fronts and defend our position on this matter) may be expressing their inner feelings about it being a battlefield. A reply that is entirely appropriate in a social setting may be regarded as offensive in a work environment.
*   **Using jargon**. The use of jargon can sometimes be an unconscious attempt to prevent communication and understanding – after all, if you do not understand what I am talking about you cannot possibly do my job! More often it is the failure to use the feedback (or lack of it) to modify what is being said to the level of understanding of the listener.
*   **Using formal or informal styles in the wrong settings**. People speak differently to their friends than to colleagues or to people at work with whom they have an unequal power relationship. Generally, the more formal the event, the more formal the language, and some people find it difficult to gauge the right level. Cultural factors affect the situation – what might seem excessively formal to an American may seem over-casual to someone from Japan.

More general tips for improving your skills for good interpersonal communication are given in Box 3.3.

Box 3.3: Skills for good interpersonal communication[13]

*   Listen with genuine interest
*   Create a conducive environment
*   Be encouraging
*   Show understanding and empathy
*   Check current understanding
*   Reflect/summarise and paraphrase answers
*   Use closed questions for exploration
*   Use open questions for clarification
*   Adopt a similar language and avoid jargon
*   Use plural pronouns to indicate partnership
*   Be provisional rather than dogmatic
*   Be descriptive not judgemental
*   Comment on the issues rather then personalities
*   Encourage eye contact
*   Give information in clear simple terms and use repetition
*   Check understanding
*   Use silence

The difference between hearing and listening – use active listening

The quality of attention that you bring to the mentoring session is achieved by a concentrated form of listening. There is a great deal of difference between *hearing* and *listening*. Hearing is a passive activity, while listening is active and requires you to *show* that you have been listening. There is a real difference between the listening that takes place with a patient when taking a case history, and the kind of listening you will need when helping a colleague to reflect on their situation. When taking a case history you are assessing what the patient says with a view to making a diagnosis. The first step with a mentee is to enable them to express themselves fully and feel understood. This process consists of reflecting back what has been said, paraphrasing and summarising at frequent intervals.

Only when someone feels certain that they are understood will they proceed to share their thoughts and feelings. That should help the mentee to off-load worries and problems and gets rid of thoughts that are blocking thinking about the future and drawing up plans for action.

Exploring

Try to use open questions to expand the conversation and encourage the other person to describe information and explore or reflect on their feelings. Avoid using 'Why?' questions as they tend to trigger defensive responses. Instead, ask 'What?,' 'How?' and 'When?' to draw the mentee out.

Creating rapport[13]

Rapport is the process of building and sustaining a relationship of mutual trust and understanding. It is the ability to relate to others in a way that makes people feel at ease. When you have rapport with someone you feel at ease, conversation flows and silences are easy. It is the basis of good communication and is a form of influence. It is a major component of listening, when the whole body indicates interest in what the other person is saying.

Building rapport is a technique described and practised in Neuro-Linguistic Programming (NLP), which is the study of what works in thinking, language and behaviour. You might use NLP to help you plan for your or your mentee's learning needs. NLP is based on a simple model of goal achievement set out as four stages:

- decide what you want
- do something
- notice what happens
- be flexible – be prepared to change.[14]

Some tips for the mentor in creating rapport and relationship building.[13]

- You should be aware of yourself and your 'body language'. Make a conscious effort to match or mirror as many of the other person's characteristics as possible: posture and the position of your body, legs, arms, hands and fingers, and how your head and shoulders are held, expression.

- Ensure that you make and keep eye contact.
- Voice – think about the pace, volume and intonation of your voice. Listen to the type of words being used by your mentee. Try to use a similar voice and words.
- Create an environment that facilitates rapport and easy conversation, for example seating position, dress, décor of room, etc.
- Be friendly and attentive, and adopt an informal style.
- Use plural pronouns to indicate partnership as appropriate, though not to imply that you as mentor are taking responsibility for the mentee's action.
- Make comments that are provisional rather than dogmatic, inviting discussion. Comment on the problem rather than make judgements.
- Ask open rather than closed questions.
- Listen actively and reflectively.
- Pick up and follow themes that the mentee introduces.
- Use clear, relevant and brief communication, rather than rambling anecdotes. It is the mentee's agenda that is important in the mentoring session. The mentor should resist any temptation to indulge themselves by enjoying reciting their own experiences for their own benefit.
- Use self-disclosure about your own fears or experiences to establish trust and common ground (but limit the extent as the self-disclosure is not to satisfy your need to unburden yourself).
- Learn to recognise and interpret and use your own feelings so that you do not relay these inappropriately to the mentee.

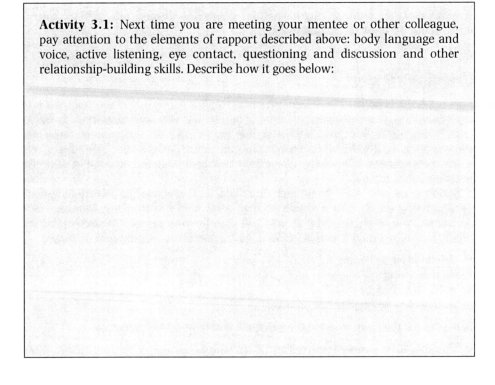

Activity 3.1: Next time you are meeting your mentee or other colleague, pay attention to the elements of rapport described above: body language and voice, active listening, eye contact, questioning and discussion and other relationship-building skills. Describe how it goes below:

Helping people out of their 'comfort zone'

As a mentor, you will want to move your mentee or others out of their usual ways of interacting with people and undertaking tasks so that they can explore new experiences and reactions. In a comfort zone, the person feels comfortable and competent.

- The aspects of everyday life feel familiar and certain.
- Work is controllable and predictable.
- There is no threat to their self-esteem or identity.
- The person has a sense of belonging.

However, people generally do not need to learn new things in their comfort zone and therefore are unlikely to change. If you push them too far they may panic and 'freeze' and will be unlikely to learn much from the experience except how to avoid it happening again. The best approach is to help people out of their comfort zone, but not into a panic zone, by encouraging them into the 'discomfort' zone instead. It is in the discomfort zone that people are most likely to change and learn how to do things differently.

To encourage people to leave the comfort zone you need to help them to feel 'safe'. You might do this by creating a compelling and positive vision together of how things could be, and discussing the systems and structures of support that exist. You can help your mentee to feel safe by creating the right supportive environment and culture where they will not be blamed for minor mistakes. Take one of their 'hot' issues and ask them to analyse their current situation from another perspective, such as that of a senior or junior colleague or patients and their carers. Discuss what training might be helpful and how they might access it. Think of positive role models that might help them visualise their way forward.

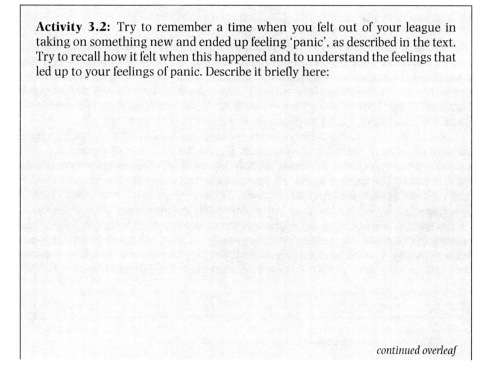

Activity 3.2: Try to remember a time when you felt out of your league in taking on something new and ended up feeling 'panic', as described in the text. Try to recall how it felt when this happened and to understand the feelings that led up to your feelings of panic. Describe it briefly here:

continued overleaf

Then consider what you might have done differently in tackling that new area so that you experienced 'discomfort' rather than 'panic'. Describe up to three actions you could have taken instead:

-

-

-

Using the JoHari window model[10,15]

The JoHari window is a useful model for thinking about communication. It will help you to understand the function of feedback and way you and your mentee relate to each other through your interpersonal activity, identifying strengths and learning needs. Figure 3.2 illustrates the concept. The four panes of the 'window' or four quadrants, represent how relationships are built up by an accumulation of information from 'self' and 'others' – in this case you as the mentor and your mentee.

Consider the crossed lines that separate the four quadrants as if they can be moved to vary the size of the four quadrants in Figure 3.3 to those of Figure 3.2. The horizontal line represents 'exposure' (that is, extent of self-disclosure by mentee). By such exposure the mentee opens up, shares ideas and information, admits mistakes and talks about their feelings and opinions. As they increase exposure, their 'façade' decreases, but the 'blind-spot' may increase through less time being given to feedback.

The vertical line in Figure 3.3 represents the mentee seeking feedback. By this, the mentee asks for and encourages or allows receipt of feedback given in an open and supportive way. Used alone, focusing on feedback may increase the façade as it allows less time for 'exposure', for the mentee to disclose their feelings and fears.

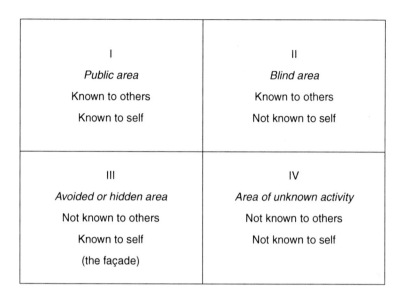

Figure 3.2:   JoHari window.

In a new relationship between mentor and mentee, the area in quadrant I is small and quadrant III is large as in Figure 3.3.

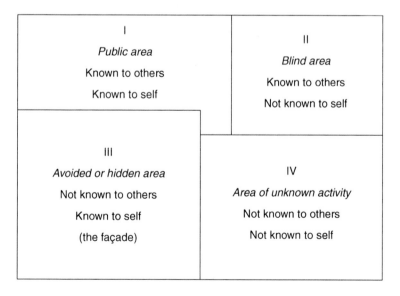

Figure 3.3:   JoHari window for new relationships.

As a mentor gets to know their mentee better, quadrant III shrinks and quadrant I enlarges. Poor communication between mentor and mentee inhibits the enlargement of quadrant I. The quadrants on the right, especially quadrant II, are susceptible to feedback from you and others, and reducing this area increases the mentee's awareness of their strengths and learning needs.

Challenge from you or your mentee's colleagues or other external factors reduces the size of quadrant IV and increases the sizes of quadrants I and II. A person's internal monitoring also helps to reduce the size of quadrant IV, so that their qualities, skills or abilities in this area can become uncovered and recognised, then moved to quadrants I or III.

There is universal curiosity about quadrants III and IV, but this is held in check by custom, social training and fear of what might be revealed. Mentors and mentees need to be sensitive about the covert content of the blind-spot, the façade and the hidden area in quadrants II, III and IV, and respect each others' privacy about information kept hidden for reasons of social training or custom.

As you try to build relationships with your mentee(s) to increase the effectiveness of your inter-relationship, the JoHari window model might help to explain why some mentor–mentee pairs have communication difficulties or are labelled poor communicators, or worse still, why the relationship becomes dysfunctional. Up to a point, the larger the area called the arena in the top left quadrant in Figure 3.3, the more productive the relationship is likely to be.

You might categorise your mentee into one of four *types* of people using this JoHari window model.

*   **Type A**: little exposure, little feedback seeking. These type of people are often perceived as withdrawn, aloof or impersonal, where the unknown square is the largest. This may induce resentment in others who may take the behaviour personally. It is common in large bureaucratic organisations.
*   **Type B**: increased feedback seeking, little exposure. These people decrease the information about themselves available to others, while requiring more from others, either through fear or a wish for power or control. Others may react by withdrawing trust or becoming hostile.
*   **Type C**: increased exposure, neglect of feedback. These people are oblivious to the impact they have on others. They have a large blind-spot as the opportunity for feedback is rare. They may be confident of their own opinions and insensitive, with little concern for the feelings of others. Listeners may become angry and reluctant to tell them anything.
*   **Type D**: balanced. These people have a large arena, as feedback seeking and exposure behaviours are well used. They are open and candid. Initially others may be put on the defensive, but once these people are seen as genuine, then productive relationships can follow. They induce an open, balanced response in others.

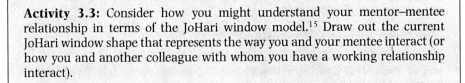

Activity 3.3: Consider how you might understand your mentor–mentee relationship in terms of the JoHari window model.[15] Draw out the current JoHari window shape that represents the way you and your mentee interact (or how you and another colleague with whom you have a working relationship interact).

What type of person are you, according to your descriptions of different types of people given above? What might you do to increase self-disclosure and feedback for yourself? Or for your mentee? Describe your 'category' and that of your mentee, and add your brief reflections here:

• Me

• My mentee

Building trust and relationships

By establishing a good relationship and mutual trust between yourself and your mentee, you are more likely to find them receptive to new ways of thinking. Trust requires two things: competency and caring. Competency alone or caring by itself will not create trust. Scholtes[16] believes that if you think someone is competent, but you do not think that they care about you or the things that are important to you, you will respect them but not necessarily trust them. On the other hand, if you think someone cares about you but you do not feel they are competent or capable, you will have affection for that person but not necessarily trust them to do the job in hand.

You can encourage people to trust you if you:

• do what you say you will do and do not make promises you cannot or will not keep
• listen to people carefully and tell them what you think they are saying. People trust others when they believe that they understand them

- understand what matters to people. People trust those who they believe are looking out for their best interests.

You can encourage good relationships with people if you:

- are able to talk to each other and are willing to listen to each other
- respect each other and know how to show respect in ways that the other person wants
- know each other well enough to understand and respect the other person's values and beliefs
- do not hide your shortcomings. This may improve your image but does not build trust
- do not confuse trustworthiness with friendship. Trust does not automatically come with friendship
- tell the truth! Be honest.

Activity 3.4: Reflect on the extent of the trust there is between you and your mentee (or another colleague if you do not have a mentee at present). What has led to that trust being created? What have you done to create or sustain that trust? List your behaviour and actions or omissions below. How has your mentee contributed to evolving trust between you? Note down your thoughts on the part your mentee has played too.

- How I have behaved:

- How my mentee has behaved:

Giving constructive feedback[17]

Constructive feedback is the art of holding conversations with others about their performance, and it has two elements: it should contain enough specific detail and advice to enable the recipient to reflect and enhance their practice and it should be positive and supportive in tone. Effective feedback has an impact not only on the learning process, but also gives messages to mentees about their effectiveness and worth, and contributes to building their self-esteem.

It is important that as well as being positive in tone (for reasons of self-esteem, morale and the development of good communication skills by observation of the mentor and others), you should balance your commentary between areas to improve and feedback that is positive in content. You should aim to give feedback about the mentee's deficiencies *and* strengths. To see why this is so, consider the following model of the development of expertise in Figure 3.4.

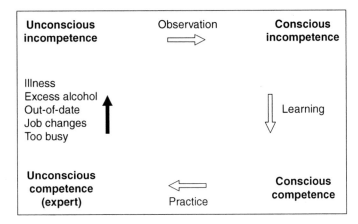

Figure 3.4: The importance of feedback in the development of expertise (competency cycle).

Starting in the top left-hand quadrant in Figure 3.4 as learners, we are blissfully unaware of our shortcomings until something happens to make us aware of them. That might be the realisation when we start working with patients that the education we had at university or college was not appropriate and that we are out of our depth. It could be a patient complaint or adverse incident or it could be feedback from a teacher.

This realisation is a painful process, often referred to as cognitive dissonance, but until we become aware we cannot start the process of learning. It is worth reminding learners that it is when you feel uncomfortable that you are just about to learn something. Too much discomfort, however, can be demotivating and some learners might give up at this stage if they feel there is too much to learn or they will never be good enough. Some feedback about the other strengths they will undoubtedly have would be supportive at this stage.

The process of learning, with all that that entails, can then proceed and we will master the new understanding, knowledge or task. We reach a stage where we know something new or know how to do something and can perform competently, so long as circumstances remain constant – as represented by the bottom right quadrant of Figure 3.4. With practice and experience we then become expert, and we can apply and modify our knowledge and skills in new situations that we may never have met before. At this stage, the bottom left quadrant, we could teach others. It is also the stage when, through familiarity, we can lose sight of our strengths, as our skills become automatic. Feedback on performance at this stage needs to include things we are good at so that we do not accept them as commonplace, we reflect on them, keep them up to date and highlight them. In some ways, feedback needs to take us from left to right across the bottom of the competency cycle to make us aware of our expertise again so that we can teach others effectively.

It is possible to move back to unconscious incompetence from the position of expertise, in the direction of the bold arrow, through dementing illness for example, or degenerative disease without insight, or even failure to keep up to date. Feedback in this position is very likely to be difficult, which is another good reason to include a reminder of remaining skills and positive attributes. (This model has some similarities with the JoHari window – *see* Figures 3.2 and 3.3 – which describes balanced communication between feedback seeking and self-disclosure to minimise the areas of hidden information in a relationship and lack of insight.)

This model provides a theoretical reason behind the observations that constructive feedback needs to contain commentary on strengths as well as things that need to be improved. It also reinforces the imperative for feedback to 'have teeth', rather than being focused exclusively on someone's strengths. The skill of the effective mentor is to find the balance between support and challenge, and the best feedback is high on both support and challenge. Figure 3.5 (opposite) describes the qualities of feedback of different dimensions.

The one golden rule for giving constructive feedback is to give positive praise of things that have been well done first. Some general rules are:

1 focus on behaviour rather than interpretation
2 give specific examples
3 aim to be descriptive or sensory based rather then interpretive, non-sensory based
4 aim to be non-judgemental rather then evaluative.

Box 3.3 gives an example of this approach as an illustration of a tutor giving feedback to a student nurse. You can read up elsewhere on different models of giving feedback.[17]

Box 3.3: Opt for a descriptive and non-judgemental approach to giving feedback

Evaluative, interpretive or judgemental	Descriptive, sensory-based
The beginning was awful, you just seemed to ignore her	At the start you were looking at the notes, which prevented eye contact
The beginning was excellent, great stuff	At the beginning you gave her your full attention and never lost eye contact – your facial expression registered interest in what she was saying
It's no good getting embarrassed when patients talk about their sexual history	I noticed you were very flushed when she spoke about her husband's impotence, and you lost eye contact ...

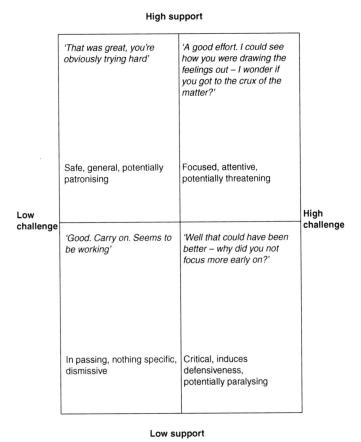

High support

'That was great, you're obviously trying hard'	*'A good effort. I could see how you were drawing the feelings out – I wonder if you got to the crux of the matter?'*
Safe, general, potentially patronising	Focused, attentive, potentially threatening
'Good. Carry on. Seems to be working'	*'Well that could have been better – why did you not focus more early on?'*
In passing, nothing specific, dismissive	Critical, induces defensiveness, potentially paralysing

Low challenge .... **High challenge**

Low support

Figure 3.5:   The qualities of feedback of different dimensions.

Activity 3.5: Obtain feedback from colleagues or others to whom you have given feedback recently on their perceptions of the quality of your own feedback. You could ask them to tell you specifically if you obey the general rules for giving good feedback listed above. Try to obtain such feedback from at least three sources.

- Reflect on the feedback you have heard and what you can learn about your skills in giving feedback to others.

continued overleaf

- Compare the ways in which these others have given you feedback – what made you feel good and worked well in realising your strengths and deficiencies from the way the feedback was conveyed?

- What aspects of their feedback reports made you feel bad or triggered feelings of defensiveness or worthlessness?

Managing conflict

Conflict and communication are inseparable. Communication can cause conflict: it is a way to express conflict and it is a way to either resolve it or perpetuate it. It is very often a breakdown in communication, or interpretation of that communication, that will inflame the conflict situation. It is the way in which conflicts surface and are addressed or resolved that dictate the outcome.

Conflict is part of change and improvement in the NHS and cannot be avoided. But it can be managed and it can turn out to be positive. Generally, conflicts have two elements, the relationship between the people involved and the issue that is the basis of the disagreement.

As a mentor, you should be able to intervene effectively in the early stages of conflict between you and your mentee by preventing, containing or handling it. And you should be able to discuss and advise your mentee about how to behave in any conflicts in which they are involved in the course of their work.

Techniques for resolving conflict[18] include the following.

1 Acknowledge that conflict exists. The disagreement may be fundamental to an issue or one small component.
2 Recognise potential benefits from the conflict situation: increased understanding and respect for others or achievements, exchange of views and attitudes, feelings surfacing, expression of energy and motivation, self-awareness, creativity, novel approaches, opportunities for change, full extent of diversity revealed.
3 Consider the options for handling conflict: for example, compromise, collaboration, co-operation, accommodation.
4 Distinguish between interests and positions within the conflict. This will enable you to understand why different parties disagree and reveal underlying assumptions contributing to the conflict.
5 Try using 'and' instead of 'or'. This approach may enable your mentee or others to realise that the conflict is not necessary and the seemingly 'conflicting' issues or approaches can be run together quite harmoniously.

6 Acknowledge and face up to 'cultural' differences if the conflict has its roots in deeply held values, beliefs and attitudes. Try to understand other people's perspectives and look at the situation from their viewpoint.

7 Attempt role negotiation by realising that a negotiated settlement is preferable to an unresolved argument.

8 Enable dialogue, encouraging both sides to suspend judgement while issues are discussed from all perspectives. Encourage those involved to keep to facts rather than opinions, to seek and explain differences, and view complex problems in new ways.

9 Establish 'rules' for conversation and discussion where the speaker may talk without you or others attacking or judging them. Termed 'no cross-talk', it means someone being able to share their 'experiences, concerns, feelings, opinions and hopes on a particular issue without referring to or reacting to anyone else's contribution and without evaluating what has been said'.[18]

Box 3.4 gives a checklist that may be useful at any stage of a conflict situation.

Box 3.4:   Tips for handling situations of conflict

Do	**Do not**
• try to cool down the debate in a hot conflict	• conduct your conversation in a public place
• convince parties in a cold conflict that something can be done	• leave the discussion open – create an action plan
• ensure that the issues are fully described	• finish another's sentence for them
• acknowledge emotions and different styles	• use jargon
• ensure you have a comfortable environment for any meeting	• constantly interrupt
• set a timeframe for the discussion	• do something else while trying to listen
• encourage good rapport between both parties	• distort the truth
• use names and, if appropriate, titles throughout	• use inappropriate humour

---

The main thing is to acknowledge any conflict and not to avoid or deny it. Describe the issues involved, talk about it and work through the conflict.

Activity 3.6: Think about a conflict situation involving you and another person, and consider on reflection:

- What was the cause of the conflict?

- How did you respond and what was the impact of this?

- How did the other person respond?

If there was a positive resolution to the conflict, how was this achieved and what did you learn from this that you might share with your mentee?

Reflecting on what you have just written and the approaches presented in the text what could you have done differently to avoid or minimise the conflict or speed its resolution?

Mentor's developmental behaviours

The table in Activity 3.7 demonstrates a variety of developmental behaviours that the mentor may adopt at any stage during the mentoring relationship. It can be a useful tool to use when reviewing how the relationship is progressing and reflecting on whether the meetings are proving to be beneficial to you both. If as a mentor you believe you are not utilising the most appropriate behaviours for certain situations, or the mentee is not doing so, you should talk over which behaviours are productive and which need some adaptation.

Activity 3.7: Look at the descriptions of the kind of behaviour listed below that a mentor should exhibit in mentoring sessions with their mentee. Copy the activity sheet and complete the right-hand column after each of three mentoring sessions. Write in comments to describe if you used that kind of behaviour in the mentoring session and your reflections of how using that behaviour worked out. Could you usefully take a different approach next time? Compare the three activity sheets to get a better idea of how you are progressing in developing your skills as a mentor.

Behaviour	*Your comments*
Challenging: Questioning the mentee's assumptions	
Encourage the mentee to think through them	
Guiding: Suggesting where to look for new knowledge or insights	
Pointing the mentee in the right direction	
Suggesting: 'Why don't you try this?'	
'You may find this will help'	

continued overleaf

Behaviour	Your comments
'Look at ...'	
Encouraging: Help mentee to reflect on previous achievements	
Motivate about new goals	
Build on confidence	
Stimulating: Lively discussion, share mentee's enthusiasm	
Direct the enthusiasm to where it will have the greatest impact	
Confiding: Draw on current projects the mentee is tackling	
Discuss the thinking process behind the judgements	
Share the options you could have taken	
Body language: Interested posture	
Good eye contact	

continued opposite

Behaviour	Your comments
Open	
Offer own experience: Drawing parallels with own experiences: 'When I faced a similar situation, I ....'	
Environmental factors: Comfortable setting, not across a desk	
Access to drinks and other facilities	
Protected from interruptions	
An agreed allocation time	

Dimension 2: Personal and people development: develop own and others' knowledge and practice across professional and organisational boundaries in relation to mentoring (Level 5)

Effective personal and people development

This means developing your own and mentees' knowledge and practice across professional and organisational boundaries by:

- understanding the healthcare context relevant to the mentee and making realistic allowances for problems and issues (including your and the mentee's attitudes, beliefs, learning styles, motivation, etc.) that might obstruct the application of best practice
- responding knowledgeably to competing demands within your everyday work
- understanding national and local healthcare priorities and how these are relevant to your and the mentee's circumstances

- evaluating the currency and sufficiency of your own knowledge and practice in your everyday work
- applying your own learning to future development of work, arising from undertaking your personal development plan (PDP)
- being able to recognise and acknowledge whether learning has occurred and been applied since the previous meeting and whether it has addressed the mentee's needs
- identifying when local developments and thinking may benefit the practice of others
- working with others (including your mentee) to develop, identify and implement appropriate learning opportunities within and outside work
- striving to improve learning strategies and opportunities to increase the overall learning and development of mentee(s) and others
- negotiating and encouraging goal setting and action plans with mentee
- supporting the development of a learning and development culture that encourages sharing of good practice.

Consider the extent to which you:

- have the knowledge and skills
- practise them – in your relationship with your mentee and in your everyday working life in other aspects of your job (you might substitute 'colleague' or 'member of staff' for 'mentee' in the list above).

Complete your audit checklist opposite in Table 3.2.

How expert are you? Think how expert you are for each aspect of effective personal and people development listed in the left-hand column of Table 3.2.

- Aware? If you are merely 'aware' you might be aware that the particular knowledge and/or skill is important and have undertaken some preliminary reading and learning, but are not yet confident, practised or skilled in employing that feature of effective personal and people development.
- Competent? If you are 'competent' you will have a good basic knowledge and be skilled in your own personal development and in developing a typical mentee.
- Expert? If you are an 'expert' you will have an enormous range of experience and intuitive grasp of situations. You will be able to interpret and synthesise information and handle a wide range of aspects of personal and people development in different contexts.[9]

How frequently do you use that aspect of effective personal and people development? Think how often you employ that feature of effective development with others at work. Is it at least daily or at least weekly or at least monthly? The more such knowledge and skills are part of your normal behaviour, the more likely they will feature naturally and consistently when you meet up with your mentee(s).

Make your assessment more objective: seek others' views of your competence or performance. You might simply ask someone else who knows you well to complete the audit Table 3.2 and compare your pre-completed table with their perspective of you – and, of course, discuss any differences with them so that you can learn from their input. You might seek feedback from your mentee towards the end of your mentoring relationship, or from others for whom you have a role or responsibility, such as in line management, educational supervision, appraisal or coaching.

Table 3.2: Self-check of own knowledge and skills in respect of personal and people development

Aspect of personal and people development	How expert are you? Aware? Competent? Expert?	How frequently do you use these? At least every day? Weekly? Monthly?
Understand healthcare context relevant to you and mentee		
Respond to competing demands		
Understand healthcare priorities		
Evaluate own knowledge and practice		
Apply own learning arising from PDP		
Recognise what mentee has learnt		
Identify when developments may benefit others		
Work with others to implement learning		
Strive to improve learning strategies and opportunities for others		
Negotiate goal setting, action planning, etc.		
Support development of learning culture		

Reflect on your own personal or your mentee's development

Understanding the healthcare context and priorities

One of the aims of the mentoring scheme you are part of will be to enable mentees to be more effective in their roles within the NHS. So you need to be familiar with the main strategies driving developments nationally and the local delivery plan of your trust. Find out more about any professional requirements of your mentee from their Royal College or other professional body.

Personal learning inventory

Everyone working in the NHS should have a personal development plan that they review with their manager or another colleague at least annually. So you might evaluate your own knowledge and practice and reflect on how you have applied what you have learnt in the past year at that review. You might use a personal learning inventory to reinforce your learning and reflect on your continuing professional development, what you have achieved and what you plan to learn about in the future.

Activity 3.8: Complete your personal learning inventory[20]

1 How will your recent learning influence your approach to:
   - lifelong learning?

   - professional development?

   - personal development?

2 How closely does your approach to learning match with the characteristics known to herald successful learning:[17]
   - based on what is already known

   - led by your identified learning/service development needs

   - involving your active participation

   - using your own resources

   - including relevant and timely feedback

   - including self-assessment?

3 How will your recent learning influence your leadership and/or management of others?

4 What are the most significant things you have learned from the issues explored in the period you are reviewing?

continued opposite

---

5   How will what you have learned change your behaviour?

6   What do you want to do differently in your current role?

7   How have you balanced competing demands?

8   Have you identified how what you have learnt and applied may benefit others? Describe your revised personal learning plan.

Force-field analysis[10]

Using a force-field analysis approach helps people to identify and focus on the positive and negative forces in their work and/or home lives and to gain an overview of the relative weighting of these factors. The exercise is suitable for anyone and everyone at any stage in their career. You might use it to review your current work situation or you might work with your mentee to enable them to review their own circumstances and need for development.

You and/or your mentee should draw a horizontal or vertical line in the middle of a sheet of paper. Ask your mentee to label one side 'positive' and the other side 'negative'. They should then draw arrows to represent individual positive drivers that motivate them on one side of the line, and negative factors that demotivate them on the other negative side of the line. The chunkiness and length of the arrows should represent the extent of the influence; that is, a short, narrow arrow will indicate that the positive or negative factor has a minor influence and a long, wide arrow a major effect (*see* Figure 3.6).

Your mentee should then take an overview of the force-field and consider if they are content with things as they are, or can think of ways to boost the positive side and minimise the negative factors. They can do this part of the exercise on their own, with a peer elsewhere or with you as mentor.

The analysis helps people to realise whether a known influence in their life is a positive or negative factor. For instance they may realise upon reflection that they had assumed that money in the form of a good salary was a positive motivator. But really, the wish to sustain or increase their income was a negative force on their job satisfaction due to their inability to spend time on meaningful non-pecuniary work-related activities.

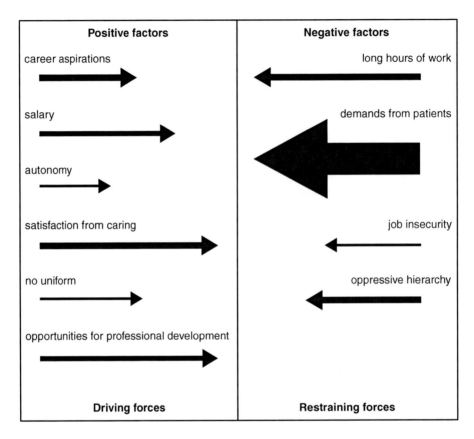

Figure 3.6: Example of a force-field analysis diagram. Satisfaction with current post as a health professional.

Activity 3.9: Draw a diagram to represent your own force-field analysis or encourage your mentee to do so in relation to their situation in the style of Figure 3.6.

continued opposite

The next step is for you/them to make a personal or organisational action plan to create the situations and opportunities to boost the positive factors in your/their life and minimise arrows on the negative side. You or your mentee could invite someone who knows them well to review the force-field analysis they have drawn and let them know honestly of any blind-spots and if they have the positive and negative influences in proportion. Analyse the forces together to determine the mentee's needs and priorities that should be addressed in planning for the change. This can be done through:

- changing the strength of a driving force: width and length of the arrows

- changing the direction of a force: switching a force to be positive rather than restraining

- withdrawing or minimising a restraining force

- adding or enlarging helping, positive forces.

Use this information for negotiating goals with your mentee and helping them to focus on action planning.

Bridging the gap

As a mentor, or enabler of your mentee, think of the gap between: 'Where you are now' and 'Where you want to be'. This gap becomes central to a planned programme of personal development and change, the nature of which depends on the various gaps identified and your/their future goals. This is a model you might use for yourself as a mentor or in your other work; or you might show your mentee as a way of helping them confront what gaps need to be filled as a pathway to attaining their goals.

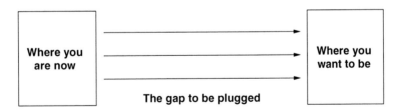

Figure 3.7:   An outline gap analysis.

Activity 3.10: Work out your own gap analysis

1   *Where you are now*: this will include a description of the important aspects of your work/home situation that are relevant to the goals you envisage and changes you want to make. It may cover your strengths and weaknesses in your current role, your experience, your transferable skills, and a review of how your current post measures up to your expectations and values.

2   *Define your future goals*: be as specific as you can be about what you want to achieve. Describe your interests, areas of work and development you'd like to be responsible for or involved in, setting you wish to work in or type of role. Outline your aspirations and preferences.

3   *Describe the gap*: compare items 1 and 2 and describe the main differences between your current state and your desired future position. Make a plan for change with timescales and milestones, so that you can monitor progress. Discuss your plan with others who know you for a reality check. Outline the opportunities that might link where you are now with your future goals.

Circles of concern and of influence

Self-awareness is vital in the process of personal change and development. One aspect of your behaviour is your own degree of proactivity – where you focus your time and energy, which influences the effects you have on others. This approach is based on Covey's model devised as a means of identifying where your energies lie, to understand what needs to happen to increase your personal effectiveness.[21]

Circle of concern: everyone has a wide range of concerns – your health, relationships, your children's future, lack of money, problems at work, the national debt, threat of nuclear war, etc. You have no real control over some of these concerns.

Reactive people focus their attention and efforts on the issues in this *circle of concern*, focusing on the weaknesses of others and on circumstances over which they have no control. This is negative in nature, as it results in blaming, defensiveness, reactive language and aggressive or passive behaviour that can lead to persecutor or victim-type reactions. Those issues that you can do something about are circumscribed in a smaller circle, called the *circle of influence* (*see* Figure 3.8). A result of being a reactive person is that those issues that are under your control and influence are neglected and underdeveloped, as your focus is elsewhere, and so your circle of

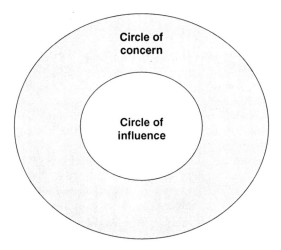

Figure 3.8: The relative positions of the Circle of concern and Circle of influence in reactive people (adapted from Covey[12]).

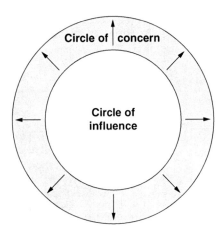

Figure 3.9: The relative positions of the Circle of concern and Circle of influence in proactive people (adapted from Covey[12]).

influence shrinks. Positive change will not occur if you are working in your circle of concern.

Proactive people focus on issues within their circle of influence; they work on things they can do something about. The nature of their energy in doing this is positive, enlarging and magnifying, and so increases the size of their circle of influence relative to their circle of concern (*see* Figure 3.9). This is adult-type behaviour, which is of a non-blaming and developmental nature. This proactive approach affects the things you have no control over within your circle of concern by enabling you to genuinely and peacefully accept those problems and issues while focusing your efforts on things you can affect. So you can learn to live with the issues in your circle of concern even if you do not like them.

Activity 3.11

Ask the mentee to draw a circle in which they depict all their issues of concern on a flipchart or piece of paper. The mentor contributes by probing and questioning, thereby identifying any other underlying concerns or facts. These can be added to the mentee's drawing.

The mentee can then transcribe the issues on to a second flipchart or piece of paper and differentiate them within their circle of concern and those that are in their circle of influence (as in Figure 3.8).

Once the mentee can visualise their issues on the charts of the circles of concern and influence, you can discuss the steps needed for the mentee to behave proactively. Encourage them to explore proactive language and behaviour in terms of the issues presented, and draw up an action plan.

A way of determining which circle the mentee's concerns are in, is by listening to the language used and distinguishing between 'have' and 'be'. 'Have' reflects the reactive state common to the circle of concern and 'Be' the proactive state typical of the circle of influence (*see* Table 3.3). The nature of reactive people is to absolve themselves of responsibility; they focus on others' weaknesses, and adopt the 'them and us' mentality. Proactive people are value-driven, aware of reality and know what is needed. They recognise that change starts with *them*.

Table 3.3:   Examples of issues that are reactive or proactive

Have (Reactive)	*Be (Proactive)*
• If only I had a boss who wasn't ...	• I can be a better role model ...
• If I had respect from ...	• I can be more organised or resourceful ...
• If I had a degree ...	• I can be more loving or understanding ...
• If I could just have management days ...	• I will be more diligent ...
• If the environment was more conducive ...	• I will be able to understand ...

Change[10,17]

There are lots of reasons why you or your mentee may be hesitant about changing the way you do things. People underestimate the barriers and hurdles to be overcome before change will be made and sustained. Many of the barriers are listed[22] below.

- Lack of perception of relevance of proposed change.
- Lack of resources to make change.
- Short-term outlook.
- Conflicting priorities.
- Lack of necessary skills.
- Limited evidence of effectiveness of proposed change.
- Perverse incentives.
- Intensity of personal contribution required.

- Having a poor appreciation of the need to change or considering the need to change to be secondary to other issues.
- Having a poor understanding of the proposed solutions or considering the solution to be inappropriate.
- Disagreeing about how the change should be implemented.
- Embarrassment about admitting that what you are doing could be improved.

Change will not be possible unless you, the mentee and managers of the organisation (e.g. trust or directorate, etc.) are committed to the change and prepared to alter the environment so that it is possible to make the change happen in practice.

As a mentor you need to understand how people react to change. As Figure 3.10 illustrates, people start off being taken by surprise about a change, even if they antici-pate it. There is still a shock element when it first happens and they may not be quite sure what has happened. They move from that shock to pretending it is not going to happen.[10]

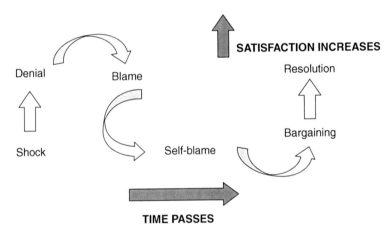

Figure 3.10: Stages in the response to change.

After the denial phase in the change process they move on to find somebody to blame for what has happened – and they tend to blame the messengers who announce the change. After the blame comes self-blame. Part of the next stage, the bargaining, is negotiating that if they do it *this* way they are going to be able to do *that*. Eventually they arrive at the resolution phase where they have accepted the change.

People pass through these different stages of change according to how they are as individuals. When change is imposed on us we are very much more resistant and move more slowly. If the effect of the change is serious, our feelings about it will be stronger and we spend longer in the phases of denial, blame and self-blame.

We need to help mentees to face up to change, by identifying the causes for dissatis-faction with the present situation, to have a clear idea of where they are heading. They should map out how to reach that target, then find their way in staged steps to measure the progress towards the target.

Teach them to recognise the roles that people play in response to change.

- The rebel – 'I don't see why I should'.
- The victim – 'I suppose you will make me, but I will drag my feet'.

- The oppressor – 'You all have to do it'.
- The rescuer – 'I will save you all from this terrible change'.

Tips for making changes

It might help to give your mentee a checklist for planning change that they can adapt to their particular situation.

- Have realistic timescales and be flexible.
- Provide clear communication about what is happening.
- Consult with all the staff, identifying all the problems as they occur.
- Plan for more resources and time than you expect to use.
- Fix interval markers of progress.
- Feed the information back to people about what is happening.
- Identify the anxieties and try to resolve them.
- Consider the effects of this change on other services and people.
- Beware of too many changes taking place at once.
- Recognise that change can be hijacked by vested interests and the direction altered.
- Be prepared to change direction if necessary.
- Beware of a lack of commitment from others.

Challenging perceptions and facilitating behavioural change[23]

When people are trying to change they experience a range of emotions and expect a range of supports to help them make the transition, as in Table 3.4.

Table 3.4:   Good practice in challenging perceptions of mentee

Emotion experienced	Support mechanism
Denial	Question the consequences of the action and options of alternatives
Anger	Acknowledge emotion, vent frustration in a measured way and introduce objectivity and others' perceptions of the situation. Discuss a positive way forward
Resistance	Individual support to identify the barriers to change and options to overcome them and achieve the change
Compromise	Identify their motivation for the change and negotiate a solution that delivers the change objectives to the individual in an acceptable way.
Acceptance	Work with them to adopt the change as habitual behaviour

Try the following Activity 3.12 as a powerful tool to move through change. It shows that you need to recognise and understand many factors from the other person's point of view in order to overcome any resistance.

Activity 3.12: Moving through change

Dissatisfaction × Vision × Capacity × First Steps ... overcomes ... Resistance
By working with the left side of the equation people will be pulled towards a change. Generally, it is better to pull people towards a change rather than push people into it. People must realise that the costs and risks of maintaining the status quo outweigh the risks and the uncertainty of making the change. Most people who have conducted successful changes stress the importance of this.

Dissatisfaction
Ask the questions:
*   how satisfied are you with the current state of things?
*   have you shared any dissatisfaction with your colleagues?
*   how is that dissatisfaction understood and experienced?

Vision
Ask the questions:
*   what do you want for your patients, yourself and your colleagues?
*   what are your values and beliefs, goals and desires?
*   what could the new system look like?

Capacity
Ask the questions:
*   what resources are needed to achieve the change? Do not forget resources such as energy and capability as well as practical things
*   how can resources be generated or shared?
*   have you shown in the past that you are willing to try out new ideas? It is most effective to test out new ideas with people who are willing to try new things
*   is there anyone that you respect both professionally and personally who has demonstrated the energy and capability to make changes? Could you get in contact with them so that you are enthused and energised by others who are similar to you?

First steps
Your mentee should identify an issue for this activity and ask the question: what first steps could I undertake which everyone agrees would be moving in the right direction?

References

1   Standing Committee on Postgraduate Medical and Dental Education (SCOPME) (1998) *Supporting Doctors and Dentists at work. An Enquiry into Mentoring.* SCOPME, London.

2   Department of Health (2003) *The NHS Knowledge and Skills Framework (NHS KSF) and Development Review Guidance – Working Draft. Version 6.* Department of Health, London.

3   Department of Health (2003) *Agenda for Change. Proposed Agreement.* Department of Health, London.

4 Chambers R, Tavabie A, See S and Hughes S (2004) Template for a competency based job description for mentors of GPs using the NHS Knowledge and Skills Framework. *Education for Primary Care.* **15**: 220–30.

5 Eraut M and du Boulay B (2000) *Developing the Attributes of Medical Professional Judgement and Competence.* University of Sussex, Sussex. Reproduced at www.informatics.sussex. ac.uk/users/bend/doh.

6 Katz AM, Siegel BS and Rappo P (1997) Reflections from a collaborative paediatric mentorship program: building a community of resources. *Ambulatory Child Health.* **3**: 101–12.

7 Galicia AR, Klima RR and Date ES (1997) Mentorship in physical medicine and rehabilitation residencies. *American Journal of Physical Medicine & Rehabilitation.* **76**: 268–75.

8 Jacobi M (1991) Mentoring and undergraduate academic success: a literature review. *Review of Educational Research.* **61(4)**: 505–32.

9 Benner P (1984) *From Novice to Expert.* Addison-Wesley, London.

10 Chambers R, Wakley G, Iqbal Z and Field S (2002) *Prescription for Learning. Techniques, Games and Activities.* Radcliffe Medical Press, Oxford.

11 Reid M and Hammersley R (2000) *Communicating Successfully in Groups.* Routledge, London.

12 Hargie ODW (1997) *The Handbook of Communication Skills* (2e). Routledge, London.

13 Tate P (2000) *The Doctors' Communication Handbook* (3e). Radcliffe Medical Press, Oxford.

14 Alder H (1996) *NLP for Managers. How to Achieve Excellence at Work.* Piatkus, London.

15 Luft J (1970) *Group Processes: an introduction to group dynamics* (2e). National Press Books, Palo Alto, California.

16 Scholtes P (1998) *The Leaders Handbook: making things happen, getting things done.* McGraw Hill, Maidenhead.

17 Mohanna K, Wall D and Chambers R (2004) *Teaching Made Easy. A Manual for Health Professionals* (2e). Radcliffe Medical Press, Oxford.

18 Elwyn G, Greenhalgh T, Macfarlane F and Koppel S (2001) *Groups: a guide to small group work in healthcare, management, education and research.* Radcliffe Medical Press, Oxford.

19 Shropshire and Staffordshire Clinical Leadership Team (2002) *Clinical Leadership Facilitators Handbook.* Shropshire and Staffordshire Strategic Health Authority, Telford.

20 Garcarz W, Chambers R and Ellis S (2003) *Make Your Healthcare Organisation a Learning Organisation.* Radcliffe Medical Press, Oxford.

21 Covey SR (1989) *The 7 Habits of Highly Effective People.* Simon and Schuster, London.

22 Dunning M, Abi-Aaad G, Gilbert D et al. (1998) *Turning Evidence into Everyday Practice.* King's Fund, London.

23 Garcarz W (2004) *Effective Mentoring for Mentors.* 4 Health Ltd, Birmingham.

4

Developing your competence as a mentor in enabling others to perform well and improve their delivery of healthcare

This chapter considers how you may develop your competence as a mentor in the other seven dimensions of the NHS Knowledge and Skills Framework (KSF) that are relevant to being a mentor.[1] As for Chapter 3, each section considers the components of the particular dimension of the KSF, and proposes tools and techniques you might use to develop your competence or show your mentee(s) to enable them to improve their performance at work.

Dimension 3: Health, safety and security: promote others' health, safety and security in relation to mentoring through risk management (Level 1)[2]

Health and safety and security is about promoting your mentee's health, safety and security by:

- being familiar with resources to which you can signpost your mentee for help or advice, e.g. occupational health, stress, financial or relationship difficulties, both within and outside the NHS
- assisting in maintaining a safe working environment for your mentee by risk management
- understanding and reporting any issues in relation to mentoring that put patient safety at risk
- being clear what constitutes mentoring and what is outside the scope of a mentor in respect of health or counselling issues
- being confident of, and abiding by, agreed ground rules for the mentoring scheme.

Consider the extent to which you:

- have the knowledge and skills
- practise them – in your relationship with your mentee and in your everyday working life in other aspects of your job (you might substitute 'colleague' or 'member of staff' for 'mentee' in the list above).

Complete your audit checklist below in Table 4.1.

How expert are you? Think how expert you are in each aspect of assisting in maintaining mentee's health, safety and security listed in the left-hand column of Table 4.1.

- Aware? If you are merely 'aware' you might be aware that the particular knowledge and/or skill is important and have undertaken some preliminary reading and learning, but are not yet confident, practised or skilled in employing that feature in assisting health, safety and security.
- Competent? If you are 'competent' you will have a good basic knowledge and be skilled in assisting with others' health, safety and security for a typical mentee.
- Expert? If you are an 'expert' you will have an enormous range of experience and intuitive grasp of situations. You will be able to interpret and synthesise information and handle a wide range of problems in assisting with others' health, safety and security in different contexts.[3]

How frequently do you use that aspect to maintain health, safety and security? Think how often you employ that feature with others at work. Is it at least daily or at least weekly or at least monthly? The more such knowledge and skills are part of your normal behaviour, the more likely they will feature naturally and consistently when you meet up with your mentee(s).

Make your assessment more objective: seek others' views of your competence or performance. You might simply ask someone else who knows you well to complete the audit Table 4.1 and compare your pre-completed table with their perspective of you – and, of course, discuss any differences with them so that you can learn from their input. You might seek feedback from your mentee towards the end of your mentoring relationship, or from others for whom you have a role or responsibility such as in line management, educational supervision, appraisal or coaching.

Table 4.1: Self-check of own knowledge and skills in respect of maintaining health, safety and security

Aspect of health, safety and security	How expert are you? Aware? Competent? Expert?	How frequently do you use these? At least every day? Weekly? Monthly?
Be familiar with network to signpost mentee for help		
Assist in maintaining a safe work environment for mentee		
Understand and report issues that put patient safety at risk		
Be clear what constitutes mentoring		
Know and abide by agreed ground rules		

Signposting mentee to other resources

If you are to sustain your role as a mentor without moving into other roles, such as counsellor, educational supervisor or pastoral support, you need to be familiar with what local resources there are within and outside the NHS, and know how your mentee may access them. Compile a logbook of resources, access arrangements and contact details, and local protocols covering the following.

- Occupational health support: for ill and distressed mentees, those with alcohol or drug misuse problems, those whose physical or mental disabilities create functional problems.
- Local process for poor or underperformance of mentee or their colleagues.
- Stress management help.
- Explicit protocols for informing others when mentor suspects or perceives that patient safety is at risk according to whether the mentee does or does not continue to work.
- Processes and resources for providing educational support for general or specific learning and development needs that are or are not recognised by mentee.
- System for allocation of resources to help the mentee address identified learning needs relating to NHS priorities, such as service development and delivery of care – what is available and contact details.
- Advice on financial difficulties.
- Counselling for relationship difficulties, within and outside work setting.
- Career information, guidance and counselling.
- Nature and frequency of ongoing support for training and development, and peer support for mentors.
- Guarantee of indemnity for mentor in the unlikely event that the mentee makes an official complaint: information about explicit limits of indemnity.
- Complaints system for mentees – nature, how to access, etc.
- Troubleshooting guide: someone or sources of help to consult if problems – relating to any/all of above.

Minimise stress[2]

Stress can be either positive or negative, depending on how you perceive it and how you react to it. If your mentee sees changes such as new regulations as challenges rather than sources of stress, they will probably find ways of managing changes to their advantage, with opportunities for learning and growth.

Stress management is considered in detail in Chapter 6 as a technique for mentees. *See* page 126 for more ideas on combating stress.

Create a safe working environment[2]

Health professionals appear to be at higher risk of work-related violence (including woundings, common assault, robbery and snatch theft) than the general population. Nurses and social workers are particularly vulnerable to aggression and violence: some have a great deal of daily one-to-one contact with patients who are mentally ill or disturbed, in circumstances where emotions run high and normally sane patients or relatives can suddenly become irrational or aggressive. Practice and community nurses, doctors, social workers and other healthcare staff who visit patients in their own homes are often unaware of danger, because their caring nature and their role as the patients' advocate makes them relatively unsuspicious of danger.

Even if they have never experienced actual violence themselves, many nurses know of vicious attacks on other health professionals and have been the victim of verbal abuse and physical threats at some time in their careers. All this may create an atmosphere of fear about their personal safety on visits to patients' homes and in other health settings where the general public has free entry.

The best way to reduce stress from aggression and violence is to prevent the episode occurring in the first place. You should discuss the following areas with the mentee who asks for your advice:

- avoiding potentially dangerous situations, especially when on visits to patients' homes
- learning how to defuse tense confrontations; being able to recognise early warning signs of aggression and being prepared to disarm anger and defuse potentially violent situations
- improving the NHS workplace so that the service provided to patients is efficient and therefore patients do not become angry because of long waits or inefficiencies
- devising a workplace policy to handle a violent or aggressive incident
- developing assertiveness and anger management skills
- learning from any violent episode and making changes to avoid a recurrence.

Verbal abuse and gesturing is thought to be at one end of a continuing spectrum that ends in physical assault. Such episodes of verbal abuse and gesturing should be treated seriously and not dismissed as trivial just because they were not accompanied by physical attack.

There should be a workplace policy in existence, with which everyone is familiar so that they know what to do to reduce the likelihood of aggression and violence flaring at work, to defuse any such incident effectively, to summon help as necessary, and to counsel and support any victim afterwards.

Unfortunately, even in reasonably happy workplaces, aggression sometimes erupts between staff. Such incidents usually arise when communication in the team is poor and the management is weak. Interpersonal conflicts can create a lot of passion and the cause of the dispute needs to be sorted out quickly and resolved before colleagues divide into two factions supporting one party or the other.

Anyone under threat of violence should try to appear confident and assertive but not aggressive, and they should be aware of the messages given out by their body language. Normally, health professionals would put patients at their ease in consultations. Defusing tension by remaining calm and unhurried is really just an extension of their normal manner.

Activity 4.1: Ask your mentee to review the safety and security arrangements of their workplace, and plan what they might do to respond if a violent episode does occur. The mentee (or you, if you are applying this activity to yourself) should circle all the preventive features currently in place in their workplace.[2]

Preventive	**In response to a violent episode**
Staff training	Support staff
Team approach	Report incident
Adequate staffing	Analyse event
Secure premises	Discuss what happened
Surgery alarms	Change systems
Good environment	Review policy
Good communication	Prosecute perpetrator of violence
Workplace policy	Review alarms
Planned interventions for different eventualities	
General awareness of danger	
Good organisation	
Culture of concern for staff	

Then consider what are the most dangerous situations for your mentee at work and what changes they can make to minimise the chances of aggression and violence arising.

Potentially threatening situations   *Intended changes*

•

•

•

•

Patient safety[5]

As a mentor, you should be aware of the seven steps to patient safety, as should anyone working in the NHS. These are:

1   build a safety culture
2   lead and support staff in patient safety matters
3   integrate risk management activity; develop systems and processes to manage risks and identify and assess things that could go wrong
4   promote reporting of incidents
5   involve and communicate with patients and the public
6   learn and share safety lessons
7   implement solutions to prevent harm, through changes to practice, processes or systems.

Your discussions with your mentee at the mentoring sessions will be likely to reinforce all aspects of this safety culture.

Being clear what constitutes mentoring

Look back at Chapter 1 for the definitions and scope of mentoring.

Activity 4.2: Describe what mentoring is about to a colleague who knows little about it and answer their questions. Check your answers against the content of Chapters 1 and 2. If you are still uncertain discuss mentoring further with the scheme organiser.

Ground rules

Look back at Chapter 2 and the section on ground rules. Undertake Activity 2.6 if you have not done it previously or with your current mentee.

Dimension 4: Service development: contribute to development of (mentoring) services (and indirectly, services for patients) (Level 3)[2]

Contribute to the development of mentoring services by:

*   encouraging reflective practice to enable the mentee to learn from their own experience
*   helping the mentee to identify their priorities for service development
*   encouraging the mentee to make improvements to services

- promoting and strengthening the mentoring programme. Alerting others to the contribution that mentoring and other learning and development can make to the development of services and the NHS.

Consider the extent to which you:

- have the knowledge and skills
- practise them – in your relationship with your mentee and in your everyday working life in other aspects of your job (you might substitute 'colleague' or 'member of staff' for 'mentee' in the list above).

Complete your audit checklist below in Table 4.2.

Table 4.2: Self-check of own knowledge and skills in respect of service development in relation to mentoring

Aspect of service development	How expert are you? Aware? Competent? Expert?	How frequently do you use these? At least every day? Weekly? Monthly?
Encourage mentee in reflective practice		
Help mentee identify priorities for service development		
Encourage mentee to improve services		
Promote and strengthen mentoring programme		

How expert are you? Think how expert you are for each aspect of effective service development in relation to mentoring listed in the left-hand column of Table 4.2.

- Aware? If you are merely 'aware' you might be aware that the particular knowledge and/or skill is important and have undertaken some preliminary reading and learning, but are not yet confident, practised or skilled in employing that feature of effective service development.
- Competent? If you are 'competent' you will have a good basic knowledge and be skilled in service development in relation to mentoring.
- Expert? If you are an 'expert' you will have an enormous range of experience and intuitive grasp of situations. You will be able to interpret and synthesise information and handle a wide range of mentoring developments in different contexts.[3]

How frequently do you use that aspect to achieve effective service development in relation to mentoring? Think how often you employ that feature of effective development with others at work. Is it at least daily or at least weekly or at least monthly? The more such knowledge and skills are part of your normal behaviour, the more likely they will feature naturally and consistently when you meet up with others who are connected with your mentoring scheme.

Make your assessment more objective: seek others' views of your competence or performance. You might simply ask someone else who knows you well to complete the audit Table 4.2 and compare your pre-completed table with their perspective of you – and, of course, discuss any differences with them so that you can learn from their input. You might seek feedback from your mentee towards the end of your mentoring relationship, or from others for whom you have a role or responsibility such as in line management, educational supervision, appraisal or coaching or mentoring scheme organiser or facilitator.

Reflective practice

Knowles has defined guidelines to encourage adult learners in reflective practice that can be generalised to a mentee.[6]

1 Establish an effective learning climate where mentees feel safe and comfortable expressing themselves.
2 Involve mentees in mutual planning of relevant methods and curricular content.
3 Trigger internal motivation by involving mentees in diagnosing their own needs.
4 Give mentees more control by encouraging them to formulate their own learning objectives.
5 Encourage mentees to identify resources and devise strategies for using the resources to achieve their objectives.
6 Support mentees in carrying out their learning plans.
7 Develop mentees' skills of critical reflection by involving them in evaluating their own learning.

Learning should be a continuous process of investigation, exploration, action, reflection and further action.

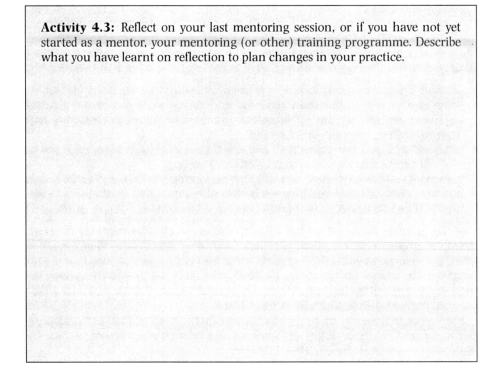

Activity 4.3: Reflect on your last mentoring session, or if you have not yet started as a mentor, your mentoring (or other) training programme. Describe what you have learnt on reflection to plan changes in your practice.

Undertake a Strengths, Weaknesses, Opportunities and Threats (SWOT) analysis: help mentee identify priorities for service development and improve services

This classic strategic planning technique can be used to analyse your or your mentee's internal capability, and to set that in relation to service development in relation to work or mentoring, from your or your mentee's perspective.

Undertake a SWOT analysis of your own performance or that of your mentee or your team or employing organisation. Work the SWOT analysis up on your own, or with your mentee, or with a group of colleagues. Brainstorm the strengths, weaknesses (or challenges), opportunities and threats of your situation.

Strengths and weaknesses of individuals might include: knowledge, experience, clinical or managerial expertise, decision making, communication, inter-professional relationships, political skills, timekeeping, organisation, expertise in teaching and research. Strengths and weaknesses for the organisation might relate to most of these aspects too, as well as resources – staff, skills or structural items.

Opportunities might relate to unexploited potential strengths, expected changes, options for career development pathways, hobbies and interests that could usefully be expanded.

Threats will include factors and circumstances that prevent you or your mentee from achieving your aims for personal, professional and team development, and improvements in patient care.

The SWOT analysis, as with so many other learning needs assessment exercises, creates opportunities to learn at the same time as undertaking the needs analysis.

Activity 4.4: The mentee should write on a single flip chart/sheet of paper so that the mentor and mentee can see all four quadrants at once.

Strengths	Weaknesses
Opportunities	Threats

continued overleaf

Each section is then completed as the mentor/mentee discuss appropriate questions, posed to explore the mentee's perceptions of environmental influences. For example:

1 Strengths – what am I good at? What factors are in my favour?
2 Weaknesses – what am I not so good at?
3 Opportunities – what's likely to be useful that I could harness? What is happening that could help me? What is new, and is it good for me?
4 Threats – what could be a threat to my/our achievements? What's new and is it bad for me?

Prioritise important factors. Draw up goals and a timed action plan.

Now compare what you produced, if working on your own, with what a colleague thought when they addressed the same task. Discuss any differences with them. Describe what you need to learn more about to address the goals that you have set for improvement of your knowledge, skills or service provision in relation to the topic(s) you have been considering.

By the end of the SWOT analysis you or the mentee should be at the stage where you can move on to consider the following.

• How can you optimise and extend the strengths identified?
• How can you minimise or overcome the weaknesses?
• How can you make most use of the opportunities?
• How can you avoid the threats or counter their effects?

Promote the impact of mentoring

Use all opportunities to let others know about the mentoring scheme and the potential benefits to the individual mentee, you as mentor, the organisation responsible for the scheme and the NHS as a whole. Contribute to any evaluation and encourage your mentees to consider becoming mentors to others.

Complete and return any evaluation forms on time. Contribute to any evaluation report of the scheme's activities. Collect information about any difficulties that obstruct the mentoring process or prevent the effectiveness of the mentoring sessions or your mentee making the most of the mentoring opportunities. Feed these back to the mentoring scheme organiser and suggest ways that the difficulties can be overcome. Join any steering group overseeing the mentoring scheme if you can, and help to influence its direction and promotion.

Dimension 5: Quality improvement: demonstrate personal commitment to quality improvement, offering others advice and support as an integral part of mentoring (Level 4)[2]

Contribute to improving the quality of your and your mentee's work by:

- demonstrating personal commitment to quality improvement
- offering your mentee advice and support in relation to quality improvement.

Consider the extent to which you:

- have the knowledge and skills
- practise them – in your relationship with your mentee and in your everyday working life in other aspects of your job (you might substitute 'colleague' or 'member of staff' for 'mentee' in the list above).

Complete your audit checklist in Table 4.3.

Table 4.3: Self-check of own knowledge and skills in respect of quality improvement in relation to mentoring

Aspect of quality improvement	How expert are you? Aware? Competent? Expert?	How frequently do you use these? At least every day? Weekly? Monthly?
Demonstrate personal commitment to quality improvement		
Offer mentee advice and support in relation to quality improvement		

How expert are you? Think how expert you are for each aspect of quality improvement in relation to mentoring listed in the left-hand column of Table 4.3.

- Aware? If you are merely 'aware' you might be aware that the particular knowledge and/or skill is important and have undertaken some preliminary reading and learning, but are not yet confident, practised or skilled in employing that feature of quality improvement.
- Competent? If you are 'competent' you will have a good basic knowledge and be skilled in quality improvement in relation to mentoring.
- Expert? If you are an 'expert' you will have an enormous range of experience and intuitive grasp of situations. You will be able to interpret and synthesise information and tackle a wide range of types of quality improvement in relation to mentoring in different contexts.[3]

How frequently do you use that aspect to achieve quality improvement in relation to mentoring? Think how often you employ that feature of effective improvement with others at work. Is it at least daily or at least weekly or at least monthly? The more such knowledge and skills are part of your normal behaviour, the more likely they will feature naturally and consistently when you meet up with others who are connected with your mentoring scheme.

Make your assessment more objective: seek others' views of your competence or performance. You might simply ask someone else who knows you well to complete the audit Table 4.3 and compare your pre-completed table with their perspective of you – and, of course, discuss any differences with them so that you can learn from their input. You might seek feedback from your mentee towards the end of your mentoring relationship, or from others for whom you have a role or responsibility, such as in line management, educational supervision, appraisal or coaching, or mentoring scheme organiser or facilitator.

Quality improvement[7]

Box 4.1 illustrates Deming's 14 points[8] that are crucial to quality improvement. The focus is to engender quality in service provision by valuing the contributions of individuals and teams, and by linking the taking of responsibility for learning to do things better directly to service improvement and increased patient or user satisfaction.

NHS organisations should be explicit about these messages and expectations. It is not realistic to assume that all healthcare workers feel a pride in what they do without any direction or guidance. Healthcare organisations now have the clinical governance framework for that direction but it is not enough on its own. It needs a process for ownership throughout the organisation, continuous learning and development to support it.

Box 4.1:   Quality improvement in a learning organisation: Deming's 14 points[8]

Deming's 14 points
1   Create constancy of purpose
2   Adopt the new philosophy
3   Cease dependence on inspection
4   Cease awarding business on price alone
5   Improve continuously and forever
6   Institute training and retraining on the job
7   Adopt and institute leadership
8   Drive out fear
9   Breakdown barriers between staff
10 Eliminate slogans and targets from the workforce
11 Eliminate numerical quotas and goals
12 Remove barriers that rob people of pride in their work
13 Institute a vigorous programme of education and self-improvement
14 Put everyone in the organisation to work on the transformation.

You might refer to Deming's points in justifying how you approach quality improvement in your own appraisal portfolio or to help your mentee increase their understanding of quality.

Organising 360° feedback[9]

As a mentor, you might recommend 360° appraisal to your mentee as a multi-source feedback tool that provides individuals with performance feedback from their peer group, managers, staff members, working partners and sometimes patients as well. The tool collects together perceptions from a number of different participants as in Figure 4.1.

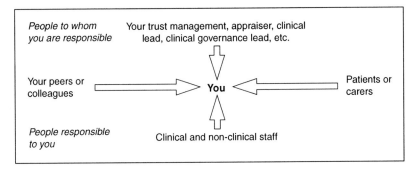

Figure 4.1:   360° feedback.

The wider the spread of people giving feedback, the more rounded the picture. Each individual gives a feedback questionnaire to at least three people in each of the groups above. An independent person then collects and collates the questionnaires and discusses the results with the individual. The main disadvantage of this method is that it can sometimes be spoilt by malicious comments against which individuals cannot readily defend themselves.

The NHS Modernisation Agency's Leadership Centre provides a model for a 360° assessment process. For further information about the tool and how to access it go to the website: www.nhsleadershipqualities.nhs.uk/assessment.asp

Significant event auditing[9,10]

Significant event auditing is a structured approach to reviewing events that have occurred at work or in your practice. Such events might be in any area of work: prevention, acute care, chronic disease, organisation or management. Significant event auditing can be a positive developmental process and is ideally suited to improving quality. You should discuss its importance in quality improvement with your mentee.

Think of an incident where a patient or you experienced an adverse event. This might be an unexpected death, an unplanned pregnancy, an avoidable side effect from prescribed medication, a violent attack on a member of staff, or an angry outburst in public by you or a work colleague. You can review the case and reflect on the sequence of events that led to that critical event occurring. It is likely that there were a multitude of factors leading up to the significant event. You should take the case to a multidisciplinary meeting to reflect and analyse what were the triggers, causes and consequences of the event. Complete the significant event audit cycle by planning what individuals or the practice as a whole might do to avoid a similar event happening in future. This might include undertaking further learning and/or making appropriate changes to the practice or your systems.

Some significant events are adverse incidents. These are events where something has clearly gone wrong, and there is a need to establish what happened, what was preventable and what changes are needed. Some adverse incidents reveal only minor risks or ones that would occur extremely infrequently and will be judged by the team as not requiring any changes. By contrast, an adverse event that is very serious, however rare, may require extensive action. In hospital settings, a range of confidential reviews such as those in maternity events, deaths and suicides provide useful occasions to review the nature of teamworking and other issues.

Risk management reporting of adverse events and near misses should be part of routine clinical governance management. In risk management reporting, there should be an easily identifiable route for action that should include:

- identifying and recording the adverse incident or near miss
- reporting to an overall monitoring body in the workplace or organisation
- analysis of the incident
- grouping together of any similar occurrences to determine any trends
- discussion of any necessary changes with the people involved
- implementing any changes necessary.

To carry out a significant event audit, a group of people who were involved in the event should meet to allow shared analysis and implementation of any necessary changes. They should be agreed on a review of the event with a no-blame attitude, and mutual trust and respect for each other. Confidentiality rules must be set out right from the start. If the patient or the participants in the care of the patient are identifiable (and they usually are), then all must be agreed on confidentiality about what is discussed and any reporting must be anonymised, so that no patients can be identified in any public document. Significant event audit uses teamworking to highlight any problems with the relationships between colleagues and staff, and to provide agreed solutions that can be implemented.

The members of the group discuss the events and some or all of the following:

- the management of the event
- any opportunities for prevention
- the follow-up
- the implications for the relatives and the community
- the actions of the clinical and non-clinical members of the team
- what action should be taken as a result of the review
- how the actions (if required) will be evaluated or monitored once put into practice.

Steps of a significant event audit

- **Step 1**: Describe who was involved, what time of day, what task/activity, the context and any other relevant information.
- **Step 2**: Reflect on the effects of the event on the participants and the professionals involved.

- **Step 3**: Discuss the reasons for the event or situation arising with other colleagues; review case notes or other records.
- **Step 4**: Decide how you or others might have behaved differently. Describe your options for how the procedures at work might be changed to minimise or eliminate the event from recurring.
- **Step 5**: Plan changes that are needed, how they will be implemented, who will be responsible for what and when, and what further training or resources are required. Then carry out the changes.
- **Step 6**: Re-audit later to see whether changes to procedures or new knowledge and skills are having the desired effects. Give feedback to the practice team.

See Activities 6.10 and 6.11 for a choice of exercises involving a significant event audit of stressful situations at work or out of work time.

Dimension 6: Equality, diversity and rights: enable others to exercise their rights and promote equal opportunities and diversity through mentoring (Level 3)[2]

Contribute to the promotion of people's equality, diversity and rights by:

- understanding the principles of equal opportunity and demonstrating best practice
- being aware of your *own* values, beliefs and attitudes and seeking to use these in a constructive manner principally, but not exclusively, in the interests of the mentee
- making evaluations and providing feedback that is free of bias and prejudice
- being open and transparent in dealings involving the mentee
- maintaining confidentiality unless required by duty or statute to do otherwise.

Consider the extent to which you:

- have the knowledge and skills
- practise them – in your relationship with your mentee and in your everyday working life in other aspects of your job (you might substitute 'colleague' or 'member of staff' for 'mentee' in the list above).

Complete your audit checklist overleaf in Table 4.4.

   How expert are you? Think how expert you are for each aspect of promoting people's quality, diversity and rights in relation to mentoring listed in the left-hand column of Table 4.4.

- Aware? If you are merely 'aware' you might be aware that the particular knowledge and/or skill is important and have undertaken some preliminary reading and learning, but are not yet confident, practised or skilled in employing that feature of promoting people's equality, diversity and rights.
- Competent? If you are 'competent' you will have a good basic knowledge and be skilled in promoting people's equality, diversity and rights in relation to mentoring.
- Expert? If you are an 'expert' you will have an enormous range of experience and intuitive grasp of situations. You will be able to interpret and synthesise information, and handle promoting people's equality, diversity and rights in different contexts.[3]

Table 4.4: Self-check of own knowledge and skills in respect of promoting people's equality, diversity and rights in relation to mentoring and other work settings

Aspect of equality, diversity, rights	How expert are you? Aware? Competent? Expert?	How frequently do you use these? At least every day? Weekly? Monthly?
Understand principles of equal opportunity and demonstrate best practice		
Use awareness of your *own* values, beliefs and attitudes in a constructive manner		
Make evaluations and provide feedback free of bias and prejudice		
Be open and transparent in dealings involving the mentee		
Maintain confidentiality unless required to do otherwise		

How frequently do you promote people's equality, diversity and rights in relation to mentoring and other work settings? Think how often you employ that feature of promotion with others at work. Is it at least daily or at least weekly or at least monthly? The more such knowledge and skills are part of your normal behaviour, the more likely they will feature naturally and consistently when you meet up with others who are connected with your mentoring scheme.

Make your assessment more objective: seek others' views of your competence or performance. You might simply ask someone else who knows you well to complete the audit Table 4.4 and compare your pre-completed table with their perspective of you – and, of course, discuss any differences with them so that you can learn from their input. You might seek feedback from your mentee towards the end of your mentoring relationship, or from others for whom you have a role or responsibility, such as in line management, educational supervision, appraisal or coaching, or mentoring scheme organiser or facilitator.

Equal opportunities and valuing diversity

The principle of equal opportunity should apply to employment, training, education, and the provision of goods, facilities or services. The principle of equal treatment guarantees freedom from discrimination on the grounds of sex, pregnancy, marital status, family status and gender reassignment.[11]

Value diversity – for it is the contrast and differences in views, style, attitudes, ethnic origins, life experiences and personality between people that provides energy and ideas. Exposing elements of diversity can be potentially threatening, as people fear that elements of themselves they would rather keep secret may be exposed (look back at the thinking around the façade and blind area in the JoHari window model on page 49). So be sensitive to diversity.

Bringing out the feelings

Look back at page 82 if you want to reflect further on how being more aware of how your own values, beliefs, attitudes and prejudices could influence your relationships with others should help you guard against such effects.

Activity 4.5: You need to establish with your mentee that it is acceptable to talk about feelings. To do that successfully, look at ways that feelings can be discussed. To initiate a discussion you might introduce a topic by writing it down on a piece of paper positioned between you. Ask your mentee to jot down their reactions to the topic under the headings:

- perceptions
- feelings
- thoughts
- behaviour.

Under *perceptions*, ask your mentee to describe both their own and other people's perceptions of the issues relating to the chosen topic.

Ask them to describe under *feelings*:
- how they have felt in the past
- what other feelings that produced
- how they feel about that now.

Under *thoughts*, ask them:
- what the things they have observed mean
- what they can learn from them
- whether there were any surprises.

Under *behaviour*, ask:
- what are you going to do as a result of your conclusions so far?
- how can you apply what you have learned?
- what are the risks of acting on your insights?
- how can you use the insights to your advantage?
- what other options do you have?
- will you do anything differently as a result of the mentoring session?

Giving effective feedback

Look back at page 53 to remind yourself of the principles and practice of giving constructive and fair feedback that is free of bias and prejudice.

Being open and transparent

Turn back to page 51 to reflect further on how to establish trust and build open and transparent relationships with your mentees, or other colleagues.

Maintaining confidentiality

One of the basic ground rules between you and your mentee will be to agree the confidential nature of the mentoring discussions, which will help to build trust. Your mentee should become increasingly trusting as they depend on you to keep their confidences, especially if you work in the same workplace or are in contact with other people the mentee may be talking about. But there are limits to confidentiality that should be explicit within the ground rules.

As a mentor, you would be especially worried about a mentee who is under-performing in some significant way(s), and appears to have no insight into their weaknesses and no plans to improve. The mentor and mentee should recognise that as professionals working in the NHS, they must protect patients when they believe that a colleague's health, conduct or performance is a threat to patients. This is clearly laid out in the Department of Health and the GMC's joint guidance on appraisal on their website www.gmc-uk.org/revalidation/index.htm and is generalisable to other professions. Therefore, if as a result of the mentoring process you believe that the activities of the mentee are such as to put their patients at risk and they refuse to seek help, and continue to work, then the mentoring process should be stopped and appropriate action taken.

Such action will depend on the mentee's post and responsibilities, but may include informing and providing evidence to their professional body, or a senior person in their employing organisation. There is nothing that can override your basic professional obligation to protect patients. You may wish to discuss the problem with the organiser or facilitator of the mentoring scheme if you are puzzled as to what action to take.

Integrity

The European Mentoring and Coaching Council (EMCC) has included a statement about confidentiality as a component of its Code of Ethics, as part of its definition of the integrity and professionalism of a mentor (or coach).[12]

Box 4.2: The European Mentoring and Coaching Council definition of integrity and professionalism in its Code of Ethics[12]

The EMCC expects that the coach/mentor will:

- maintain throughout the level of confidentiality that is appropriate and is agreed at the start of the relationship
- disclose information only where explicitly agreed with the client and sponsor (where one exists), unless the coach/mentor believes that there is convincing evidence of serious danger to the client or others if the information is withheld
- act within applicable law and not encourage, assist or collude with others engaged in conduct that is dishonest, unlawful, unprofessional or discriminatory
- not exploit the client in any manner, including, but not limited to, financial, sexual or those matters within the professional relationship. The coach/mentor will ensure that the duration of the coach/mentoring contract is only as long as is necessary for the client/sponsor

continued opposite

- understand that professional responsibilities continue beyond the termination of any coach/mentoring relationship. These include the following:
  - maintenance of agreed confidentiality of all information relating to clients and sponsors
  - avoidance of any exploitation of the former relationship
  - provision of any follow-up that has been agreed to
  - safe and secure maintenance of all related records and data
- ensure that any claim of professional competence, qualifications or accreditation is clearly and accurately explained to potential clients and that no false or misleading claims are made or implied in any published material.

Dimension 7: Promotion of self-care and peer support: encourage others to promote their own health and wellbeing through mentoring (Level 1)[2]

Contribute to the promotion of mentee's health and wellbeing by:

- encouraging the mentee to promote their own current and future health and wellbeing
- being sensitive to the mentee's health concerns that may impair their performance and/or judgement.

Consider the extent to which you:

- have the knowledge and skills
- practise them – in your relationship with your mentee and in your everyday working life in other aspects of your job (you might substitute 'colleague' or 'member of staff' for 'mentee' in the list above).

Complete your audit checklist in Table 4.5.

Table 4.5: Self-check of own knowledge and skills in promotion of mentee's health and wellbeing

Aspect of health and wellbeing	How expert are you? Aware? Competent? Expert?	How frequently do you use these? At least every day? Weekly? Monthly?
Encourage mentee to promote their own current and future health and wellbeing		
Be sensitive to mentee's health problems that may impair performance and/or judgement		

How expert are you? Think how expert you are in promoting your mentee's health and wellbeing as listed in the left-hand column of Table 4.5.

- Aware? If you are merely 'aware' you might be aware that the particular knowledge and/or skill is important and have undertaken some preliminary reading and learning, but are not yet confident, practised or skilled in promoting your mentee's health and wellbeing.
- Competent? If you are 'competent' you will have a good basic knowledge and be skilled in promotion of your mentee's health and wellbeing.
- Expert? If you are an 'expert' you will have an enormous range of experience and intuitive grasp of situations. You will be able to interpret and synthesise information and promote your mentee's health and wellbeing in different contexts and circumstances.[3]

How frequently do you promote mentee's health and wellbeing? Think how often you promote your mentee's health and wellbeing or that of others at work. Is it at least daily or at least weekly or at least monthly? The more such knowledge and skills are part of your normal behaviour, the more likely they will feature naturally and consistently when you meet up with others who are connected with your mentoring scheme.

Make your assessment more objective: seek others' views of your competence or performance. You might simply ask someone else who knows you well to complete the audit Table 4.5 and compare your pre-completed table with their perspective of you – and, of course, discuss any differences with them so that you can learn from their input. You might seek feedback from your mentee towards the end of your mentoring relationship, or from others for whom you have a role or responsibility such as in line management, educational supervision, appraisal or coaching, or mentoring scheme organiser or facilitator.

Promotion of mentee's health and wellbeing

Read through the various helpful approaches in Chapter 6. These are aimed at the mentee, and you can reinforce the importance of your mentee making time and focusing energy on looking after themselves and staying healthy. They may welcome the opportunity to seek your objective input on the way they balance their work and home lives, and deal with competing priorities. You should be in a position to signpost them to other sources of help for stress and health problems (*see* page 77).

The NHS has much more emphasis on staff wellbeing these days through the Improving Working Lives (IWL) initiatives developing in every trust. So it may be worth you finding out more about how local or national IWL initiatives could help.[13] Otherwise, encourage your mentee to undertake an activity such as Activity 4.6 to review and then plan a change to their life which will boost their wellbeing.

Activity 4.6: Boost your wellbeing. Think of a new situation in your professional or personal life that has created pressure on you, e.g. a new relationship with a partner, house move or taking up a new post.

* Who initiated the situation or change?
* How did it all start?
* Who was involved?
* Who was affected by any change?
* Were there any repercussions?
* To what extent were you in control of the circumstances of the change?

Now think about 'your' approach to the change and consider your strengths, in terms of behaviours (*see* page 71). On reflection – how appropriate has your behaviour been?

Then consider how your strengths and areas for improvement could impact on the change process by completing the table below?

How could your strengths impact on the change process?	*How could your areas for improvement impact on the change process?*

Handling health problems that may impair performance or judgement

It is possible, but very unlikely, that from what you hear during your mentoring discussions you, as a mentor, may have serious concerns about the safety of patients cared for by your mentee due to their health problems. Figure 3.2 in the section on giving constructive feedback (*see* page 49) listed some health-related reasons why a professional's competence might be impaired. These include problems with misuse of alcohol or other illicit substances, mental health problems such as psychosis without insight, and severe depression.

Persuading the impaired mentee to see their own GP and follow his or her management will probably be the best course of action. Do not get involved yourself in giving health advice or treatment to the mentee.

If a situation did crop up where you became aware that patient safety was at risk from your impaired mentee and they persisted in remaining at work, you should know how to act along the lines discussed under 'Maintaining confidentiality' (*see* page 92).

Dimension 8: Partnership and support: develop and sustain partnership working with mentees and the healthcare organisation/deanery (as appropriate) (Level 1)[2]

Contribute to partnership working in relation to mentoring by:

- developing and sustaining partnership working between mentor, mentee and organisation
- fostering teamwork and good working relationships with other parts of the health service.

Consider the extent to which you:

- have the knowledge and skills
- practise them – in your relationship with your mentee and in your everyday working life in other aspects of your job (you might substitute 'colleague' or 'member of staff' for 'mentee' in the list above).

Complete your audit checklist in Table 4.6.

Table 4.6: Self-check of own knowledge and skills in respect of participating in partnership working in relation to mentoring

Aspect of partnership/ teamworking	*How expert are you? Aware? Competent? Expert?*	*How frequently do you use these? At least every day? Weekly? Monthly?*
Develop and sustain partnership working between mentor, mentee and organisation		
Foster teamwork and good working relationships with other parts of NHS		

How expert are you? Think how expert you are for each aspect of partnership working in relation to mentoring listed in the left-hand column of Table 4.6.

- Aware? If you are merely 'aware' you might be aware that the particular knowledge and/or skill is important and have undertaken some preliminary reading and learning, but are not yet confident, practised or skilled in partnership or team-working in relation to mentoring.
- Competent? If you are 'competent' you will have a good basic knowledge and be skilled in partnership or teamworking in relation to mentoring.

- Expert? If you are an 'expert' you will have an enormous range of experience and intuitive grasp of situations. You will be able to interpret and synthesise information and participate in partnership and teamworking in relation to mentoring in different contexts.[3]

How frequently do you participate in partnership working in relation to mentoring? Think how often you employ partnership working with others at work. Is it at least daily or at least weekly or at least monthly? The more such knowledge and skills are part of your normal behaviour, the more likely they will feature naturally and consistently when you meet up with others who are connected with your mentoring scheme.

Make your assessment more objective: seek others' views of your competence or performance. You might simply ask someone else who knows you well to complete the audit Table 4.6 and compare your pre-completed table with their perspective of you – and, of course, discuss any differences with them so that you can learn from their input. You might seek feedback from your mentee towards the end of your mentoring relationship, or from others for whom you have a role or responsibility such as in line management, educational supervision, appraisal or coaching, or mentoring scheme organiser or facilitator.

Working in teams[14]

You should focus on encouraging common understanding of people's roles, responsibilities and capabilities in helping others to understand the benefits of teamworking and working in partnership.

One way to help people understand more about how they perform in a certain role within a team is to use psychometric or psychological measurements or interpersonal assessment, such as the Belbin self-perception inventory.[15] Although teams are made up of individuals, each member fulfils a different role. Different situations dictate the role an individual will adopt, and in some situations roles may be duplicated or one person will play a combination of roles. All roles will be in evidence in any effective social or workgroup, although it is possible for groups to survive and achieve some of their objectives with one or more of the roles unfilled.

The eight roles identified by Belbin in a 'winning team' are:

- **chairman or co-ordinator**: co-ordinating leadership, clarifies goals and priorities
- **plant**: generator of ideas, solves difficult problems
- **monitor or evaluator**: 'sifter' of ideas, sees all options, analyses, judges likely outcomes
- **teamworker**: looks after internal relationships, listens, handles difficult people
- **resource investigator**: looks after the external relationships, networking, explores new possibilities
- **company worker**: loyal to the group, organises, turns ideas and plans into practical forms of action
- **shaper**: challenges, pressurises, finds ways round obstacles
- **completer/finisher**: ensures tasks and projects are completed, keeps others to schedules and targets.

Activity 4.7: You might encourage your mentee to complete the Belbin inventory and find out more about the role(s) they prefer to play in a team.

Working in partnerships

People are more likely to learn about the benefits of working in partnerships and develop new meaningful partnerships themselves by observing others as successful role models. The positive features of partnerships that are most likely to be successful are listed below. Good partnerships between different disciplines or the NHS and other organisations, such as those in the voluntary sector or social services, depend on creating trust, mutual respect and joint working for common goals:[14]

- a written memorandum of partnership
- a joint strategy with agreed goals and outcomes
- widespread support by individuals working within the partnership and their organisations
- clear roles and responsibilities with respect to joint working
- shared decision making on partnership matters
- each partner has different attributes which fit well with the other partner
- the partnership benefits all contributors
- the whole partnership is greater than the sum of the components
- each partner makes a 'fair' investment in the partnership – and the risk/benefit balance is fair between partners
- partners trust each other and are honest over partnership matters
- partners appreciate, respect and tolerate each others' differences
- there is a common understanding about language and communication.

Activity 4.8: Agree a task with your mentee that will require them to work in partnerships with others and then analyse how that partnership was created and sustained. Try to arrange it so that the task requires the mentee to gather information that is only available elsewhere, so that seeking it introduces them to other sectors, including health, and non-health settings such as social care, higher education, housing or transport.

Activity 4.9: Arrange with your mentee that they will shadow someone who holds a post to which they aspire or would benefit from knowing more about, so that they can get real insights about another job or sector or type of work. Discuss what they have learnt after the shadowing session(s) have taken place and the insights they have gained in respect of partnership or teamworking, and how this will influence their career or development plan.

Dimension 9: Leadership skills: lead others in the development of knowledge, ideas and work practice as integral part of mentoring (Level 2)[2]

Contribute to the development of leadership by:

- leading and inspiring your mentee in the development of knowledge, ideas and work practice
- recognising your own leadership skills and those of others.

Consider the extent to which you:

- have the knowledge and skills
- practise them – in your relationship with your mentee and in your everyday working life in other aspects of your job (you might substitute 'colleague' or 'member of staff' for 'mentee' in the list above).

Complete your audit checklist below in Table 4.7.

Table 4.7: Self-check of own knowledge and skills in respect of leadership in relation to mentoring and everyday work

Aspect of leadership skills	How expert are you? Aware? Competent? Expert?	How frequently do you use these? At least every day? Weekly? Monthly?
Lead and inspire your mentee in development of knowledge, ideas and work practice		
Recognise your own leadership skills and those of others		

How expert are you? Think how expert you are for each aspect of the development of leadership in relation to mentoring listed in the left-hand column of Table 4.7.

- Aware? If you are merely 'aware' you might be aware that the particular knowledge and/or skill is important and have undertaken some preliminary reading and learning, but are not yet confident, practised or skilled in developing leadership.
- Competent? If you are 'competent' you will have a good basic knowledge and be skilled in leadership in relation to mentoring.
- Expert? If you are an 'expert' you will have an enormous range of experience and intuitive grasp of situations. You will be able to interpret and synthesise information and provide leadership in relation to mentoring in different contexts.[3]

How frequently do you provide leadership in relation to mentoring or your everyday work? Is it at least daily or at least weekly or at least monthly? The more such knowledge and skills are part of your normal behaviour, the more likely they will feature naturally and consistently when you meet up with others who are connected with your mentoring scheme.

Make your assessment more objective: seek others' views of your competence or performance. You might simply ask someone else who knows you well to complete the audit Table 4.7 and compare your pre-completed table with their perspective of you – and, of course, discuss any differences with them so that you can learn from their input. You might seek feedback from your mentee towards the end of your mentoring relationship, or from others for whom you have a role or responsibility such as in line management, educational supervision, appraisal or coaching, or mentoring scheme organiser or facilitator.

Leadership

It is important that leaders invest time and effort in mentoring. In these target-driven times in the NHS, leaders may say 'I don't have time to be a mentor' (or be mentored). By ignoring this they are missing a powerful and rewarding tool.

Leaders are those people in your organisation who have responsibility for developing vision, strategic planning, organisational performance, redesign and extension of services, service quality and workforce development, as in Box 4.3.

Box 4.3: Leaders in health and social care[16]

Leaders work with others to visualise how change could make an improvement, they create a climate in which the plans for change are developed and widely accepted and they stimulate action to achieve the change.

Leaders are involved in developing awareness that change is necessary, in visualising the nature of change, in progressing the journey from one state to another and in taking ownership of the change so that it becomes the new 'normal' state.

People-oriented leadership styles concentrate on good working relationships and the wellbeing of staff. Task-oriented leadership styles focus on setting goals and planning activities to ensure that the task is completed successfully.

People usually become leaders by being appointed to a leadership role. Sometimes they attain leadership positions because they have a personal interest in an initiative. Another alternative is when a concerned and able person steps forward to fill a vacuum in an area of activity. At other times, an unwilling leader has gained that role because others have thought they are right for the job and encouraged them to take it on, or thrust it upon them.

Activity 4.10: How do people become leaders? Think about leaders you know in different areas of work. Make a note of four ways that people you know have become leaders.

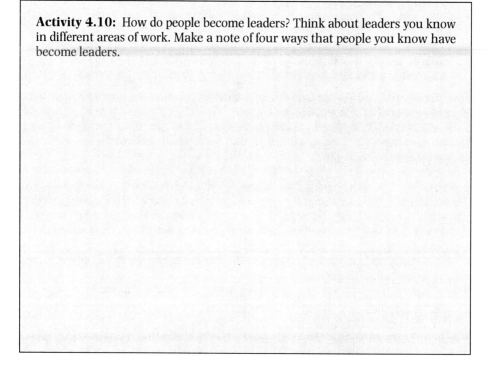

One formulation of the leadership role is: to direct and co-ordinate the work of others to build, support and work with teams, to work effectively as part of a team, and to negotiate and consult effectively. This type of leadership emphasises the 'democratic' concept of team leadership. A team leader with a democratic style enables a team to function well and encourages rather than imposes change.[7]

Leadership styles vary greatly, ranging from authoritarian to developmental (*see* Box 4.4). The categories are not mutually exclusive, and each style is relevant in the appropriate context.

Box 4.4: Leadership styles[17]

1 **Authoritarian**: giving clear directions for specific tasks
2 **Authoritative**: stating broad objectives and delegating the detailed execution to others while accepting responsibility for the outcome
3 **Democratic**: encouraging participation to secure the benefit of the expertise of all team members
4 **Task-oriented**: focusing on the task in hand and requiring a high standard of task accomplishment, regardless of other considerations
5 **Developmental**: focusing on the longer-term development of members of the team as an investment in the future

---

Activity 4.11: Reflect on what type of leader you are and why. Discuss your self-analysis at your next appraisal with your line manager or appraiser, and seek their insights and suggestions as to how you might change your leadership style, if that is appropriate.

Box 4.5 includes insights from various leadership initiatives that describe the attributes of leaders in health settings.

Box 4.5: Leaders in health settings[18-20]

- Develop and articulate a vision. They understand the rationale and show how the vision can be realised. They engage people in developing the vision and reflect the vision in strategies and action
- Motivate others. They design jobs so that people perform well. They invest time and energy in supporting and listening to people. They know how to motivate people and encourage high standards
- Make decisions. They recognise that uncertainty and risk is part of decision making; they seek the views and opinions of key people and engage others in taking decisions. They are prepared to take difficult and unpopular decisions. They learn from, and monitor, the effects of previous decisions

continued overleaf

- Release others' talents. They identify and overcome barriers for individuals, teams and organisations in achieving their potential. They ensure that individuals' learning and development needs are identified and met
- Demonstrate responsiveness and flexibility. They are able to respond positively and competently to an unexpected event themselves, and develop a culture of flexibility and responsiveness in the organisation as priorities change. They recognise the pressures people are under when there is uncertainty and change
- Embody a set of values. They make the values of the organisation clear to others internally and externally, and create respect for people with whom they work, service users and members of the public. They work towards equity and access to services and are good role models themselves in terms of their conduct and personal behaviour
- Innovate. They encourage a culture where creativity and innovation are welcomed and people learn from past successes or failures. They try out new ideas from within and outside the organisation
- Work across boundaries. They are committed to working in partnership and overcoming barriers to joint working (e.g. tackling professional tribalism, different structures and cultures). They create opportunities for joint working and can negotiate with partner organisations to minimise conflicting priorities
- Demonstrate resilience and assistance. They not only demonstrate self-confidence themselves, but build confidence in individuals and teams. They develop strategies to avoid burnout in the workforce and have insight as to their own and others' strengths and weaknesses

Activity 4.12: Seek feedback from other colleagues about the nature of your leadership skills and practice. Ask them to make comments about how you are as a leader against the headings from Box 4.5. Do you:

- develop and articulate a vision?

- motivate others?

- make decisions?

continued opposite

- release others' talents?

- act in responsive and flexible ways?

- embody a set of values?

- innovate?

- work across boundaries?

- show resilience – building others' confidence?

Transactional leaders

Transactional leaders closely resemble the traditional definition of a manager. It is not unusual for transactional leaders to offer rewards to ensure tasks are completed and as a means of getting better performance from others. Their primary focus is on management tasks and 'getting the job done', rather than how people feel doing the job.

Transformational leaders

Transformational leadership raises the level of human conduct and ethical aspiration of both the leader and those being led, and thus has a transforming effect on both.

This type of leader is visionary, inspiring others to excel, ensuring that individuals' needs, and those of teams and the organisation, are considered. Transformational leaders stimulate people to think more creatively, and enable others to act and discover new ways to deal with people and situations. They are willing to take risks, to innovate and experiment with good ideas, and to challenge the system.

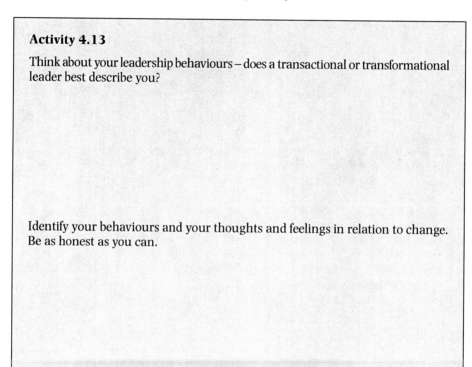

Activity 4.13

Think about your leadership behaviours – does a transactional or transformational leader best describe you?

Identify your behaviours and your thoughts and feelings in relation to change. Be as honest as you can.

And lastly ... protected time: identify and negotiate protected time to devote to the mentoring process

This tenth requirement of mentors is not a dimension within the NHS KSF, but it is a pre-requisite for a mentor to be able to devote sufficient dedicated time to their mentoring role and mentoring meetings.

A mentor should be able to demonstrate through record keeping and feedback from others that they:

• make time for the individuals whom they mentor and their follow-up meeting and plans
• take an active part in local training or support sessions, which provide peer support for mentors and others in connection with mentoring (as appropriate).

References

1   Department of Health (2003) *The NHS Knowledge and Skills Framework. Version 6.* Department of Health, London.

2   Chambers R, Tavabie A, See S and Hughes S (2004) Template for a competency based job description for mentors of GPs using the NHS Knowledge and Skills Framework. *Education for Primary Care.* **15**: 220–30.

3   Benner P (1984) *From Novice to Expert.* Addison-Wesley, London.

4   Chambers R (1998) *Survival Skills for GPs.* Radcliffe Medical Press, Oxford.

5   National Patient Safety Agency (2003) *Seven Steps to Patient Safety. A Guide for NHS Staff.* National Patient Safety Agency, London.

6   Knowles MS (1984) *Andragogy in Action: applying modern principles of adult learning.* Josey-Bass, San Francisco.

7   Garcarz W, Chambers R and Ellis S (2003) *Make Your Healthcare Organisation a Learning Organisation.* Radcliffe Medical Press, Oxford.

8   Deming WE (1986) *Out of the Crisis.* Cambridge University Press, Cambridge.

9   Chambers R, Wakley G, Field S and Ellis S (2003) *Appraisal for the Apprehensive.* Radcliffe Medical Press, Oxford.

10 Pringle M, Bradley CP, Carmichael C *et al.* (1995) *Significant Event Auditing.* Occasional Paper No. 70. Royal College of General Practitioners, London.

11 Equal Opportunities Commission (1998) *Equality in the 21st Century.* Equal Opportunities Commission, Manchester.

12 European Mentoring and Coaching Council (2004) *Code of Ethics.* European Mentoring and Coaching Council, Sherwood House, 7 Oxhey Road, Watford, Hertfordshire WD19 4QF or www.emccouncil.org

13 Improving Working Lives www.dh.gov.uk/PolicyAndGuidance/HumanResourcesAnd Training/ModelEmployer/ImprovingWorkingLives/fs/en

14 Mohanna K, Wall D and Chambers R (2004) *Teaching Made Easy. A Manual for Health Professionals* (2e). Radcliffe Medical Press, Oxford.

15 Belbin RM (1981) *Managerial Teams. Why They Succeed or Fail.* Heinemann, Oxford.

16 Martin V (2003) *Leading Change in Health and Social Care.* Routledge, London.

17 Rashid A and McAvoy P (2002) Managing to be a successful leader. *GP.* **30 September**: 40–2.

18 Frances D and Woodcock M (1996) *The Unblocked Manager.* Gower, Aldershot.

19 Scott T (2000) Clinicians in management. In: Leadership in Health; a UK Perspective on Clinical Leadership – Part 2. *Healthcare Review Online™.* **4(2)**.

20 Simpson J (2000) Clinical leadership in the UK. In: Leadership in Health; a UK Perspective on Clinical Leadership – Part 2. *Healthcare Review Online™.* **4(2)**.

5

Demonstrating your competence as a mentor

As a professional, you should be able to demonstrate your competence in the roles of your daily work – for appraisal or revalidation of your professional qualifications. If you are working as a mentor you should gather evidence that you are staying up to date and maintaining your competence as a mentor, as well as in other areas of your work. In the drive to regulate professionals' standards of practice, everyone must collect and retain information that demonstrates their current competence in their work as part of the clinical governance culture in their organisation.

Box 5.1 summarises a description of an effective mentor – but how can you demonstrate this or show that you are working towards deserving this description?

Box 5.1: Summary – being effective as a mentor

Run through the checklist below to see if you are a mentor who works effectively with individuals. Do you:

- put your main effort into trying to understand the other person? Every person is unique – respect the other person's view of the world
- develop a range of styles for working with your mentee? Do not just rely on one or two ways
- ask open questions and show you are using active listening skills?
- create a real rapport with your mentee with appropriate non-verbal communication?
- ask for feedback? Are you aware of yourself and how you appear to others?
- understand that every behaviour is useful in some way and use this knowledge?

The stages of evidence cycle

The stages of the evidence cycle for demonstrating your standards of practice or competence, and any necessary improvements in your practice as a mentor, are given in Figure 5.1. Although the five stages are shown here in sequence, in practice, you would expect to move backwards and forwards from stage to stage, because of new information or a modification of your earlier ideas. New information might accrue, which affects your mentoring methods or standards, or a critical incident or mentee complaint might occur, which causes you and others to think anew about the way you work. The arrows in Figure 5.1 show that you might re-set your target or

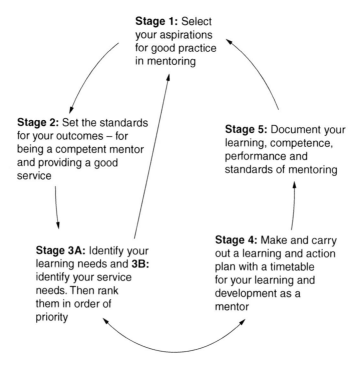

Figure 5.1:   Stages of the evidence cycle.[1,2]

aspirations for good practice having undertaken exercises to identify what you need to learn or determine whether there are deficiencies in your mentoring or day-to-day work practice.

As you start to collate information around this five-stage cycle, discuss any problems about mentoring with colleagues, experts in this area, tutors, etc. You will want to develop a wide range and depth of evidence so that you can show that you are competent in your general day-to-day work as a health professional or manager, as well as your expertise as a mentor. Box 5.2 gives a definition of competence that is applicable to staff working in health settings.[3]

Box 5.2:   Competence is defined as:

'able to perform the tasks and roles required to the expected standard'[3]

You should be able to demonstrate that you can maintain a satisfactory standard most of the time in your mentoring and everyday work. Some of the time you will be brilliant, of course! Celebrate those moments. On other occasions, you or others will be critical of your performance and feel that you could have done much better. Reflect on those episodes to learn from them.

You will need to describe the standards expected in the range of tasks and roles you undertake as a mentor, or in other areas of your work, and reference the source of standard setting. If professionals, or their organisations, are the only people involved in setting those standards, consider whether you should amend or extend the standards, tasks or roles by considering other perspectives, such as those of mentees, patients or the NHS as a whole. The European Mentoring and Coaching Council (EMCC) has set standards for a competent mentor in its Code of Ethics (*see* Box 5.3) – these might be the standard you apply to the definition of competence in Box 5.2, for example, if you endorsed the EMCC's definition.[4] Alternatively, you may base your definition of competence on the descriptions included in Chapters 3 and 4 of this book, which are based on the NHS Knowledge and Skills Framework and captured in the 'Job description of a mentor' in Chapter 7 (*see* page 139).

Box 5.3:   Description of a competent mentor[4]

The European Mentoring and Coaching Council (EMCC) Code of Ethics sets out what clients and sponsors can expect from the coach/mentor in either a coach/mentoring, training or supervisory relationship. They describe a competent coach/mentor as someone who:

(a)   ensures that their level of experience and knowledge is sufficient to meet the needs of the client

(b)   ensures that their capability is sufficient to enable them to operate according to this Code of Ethics and any standards that may subsequently be produced

(c)   develops and then enhances their level of competence by participating in relevant training and appropriate continuing professional development activities

(d)   maintains a relationship with a suitably qualified supervisor, who will regularly assess their competence and support their development.

There is a difference between being competent and performing in a consistently competent manner. You need to be motivated to perform consistently well and enabled to do so with efficient systems and sufficient resources. You will require sufficient numbers of other staff and available infrastructure for performing well in your day-to-day work, and protected time, good administrative support and training resources to perform well as a mentor, for example.

Example of evidence to demonstrate that you are a competent mentor

The following example gives an illustrative cycle of evidence you might use or adapt to enable you to gather evidence that you are performing well as a mentor. It is reproduced from: Chambers *et al.* (2004).[2] You might want to copy the example in your own mentoring practice, or adapt it and draw up your own approach to gathering evidence to show that you are a competent mentor.

Case Study: Mentoring

You have just volunteered to be a mentor because you have gained so much from being mentored yourself. You had a mentor for the first year after you qualified and again more recently. The first relationship worked well and your mentor was non-judgemental, empathetic, open and approachable. The second mentor used to unload his own problems at the end of each mentoring session and you were glad when he explained that with the changes in NHS working he just had not got time to carry on. You thought this was an excuse to save face, because it was obvious that the relationship was not working. You resolve to be as good as your first mentor.

Stage 1: Select your aspirations for good practice

The excellent healthcare mentor:

- establishes an honest and trustworthy relationship with the person being mentored
- guides the person being mentored to take up personal, professional and career development opportunities.

Stage 2: Set the standards for your outcomes

Outcomes might include:

- the way learning is applied
- a learnt skill
- a protocol
- a strategy that is implemented
- meeting recommended standards.

1   Establish a good and open relationship between both parties, by adopting formative and supportive roles.
2   The person being mentored gains new insights and perspectives and enjoys being challenged to change.

Stage 3A: Identify your learning needs

If you have not started out as a mentor and are considering it, you should do the following:

1   Reflect on the good qualities of a mentor and check the extent to which you already have those qualities by discussion with a trusted colleague or friend. Ask them if they would provide a reference for you to support your application to be a mentor, as an exercise for you to read and consider their perspectives.
2   Talk to others who are mentors: what is the time commitment, how do they deal with interpersonal conflicts, how long has the mentoring relationship lasted, how do they defuse the 'halo' effect if it happens, are they paid, and if not can the meetings be carried out in non-work time? Reflect whether you can create that spare time and maintain the degree of commitment needed over time.

3   In your discussion with the mentoring lead, find out how much training is provided or available, and what ongoing support is arranged.
4   Obtain a job description for the mentor role or ask the mentor lead to write one if none exists; make a judgement about whether you have sufficient knowledge and skills or training needs.

If you have started as a mentor already, do the following.

5   Work out a system with the lead for recruiting and supporting mentors. Ask the current person being mentored for their honest appraisal of your strengths and weaknesses as a mentor.
6   Participate in role-play exercises at mentor training and support sessions, and receive peer feedback on your attitudes and responses.

Stage 3B: Identify your service needs

Any of the needs assessment exercises in Stage 3A may also reveal service needs.

1   Ask the lead for recruiting mentors for anonymised feedback from the people you have mentored.

Stage 4: Make and carry out a learning and action plan

1   Attend training workshop for new or potential mentors.
2   Talk to established mentors and anyone who tells you that they are being or have been mentored. Find out what it is they most value about the relationship.
3   Read widely about the history and practice of mentoring in health settings and other public or commercial sectors.
4   Learn how to record and use informal feedback by discussion with others at peer group meetings.

Stage 5: Document your learning, competence, performance and standards of service delivery

1   Job description for mentor role with written reflections as to your knowledge, skills and training needs, and how they will or have been met.
2   Feedback from the person being mentored or from those mentored in the past.
3   Notes of key points and what you have learnt from recommended reading material.
4   Copy of your mentoring contract.

Case Study continued

You attend the initial training workshop and follow-up session six months later, once the mentoring is underway. You really gel with your new mentee, who would be surprised to know that she is the first person you have mentored. She particularly benefits from your skills at challenging her perceptions and perspectives and goes on to represent staff in strategic working groups, which she would not have previously dared to do.

Activity 5.1: Now you draw up your five-stage cycle of evidence to demonstrate that you are a competent mentor.

• Stage 1: Set your aspirations for good practice

• Stage 2: Set the standards for your outcomes

• Stage 3A: Identify your learning needs

• Stage 3B: Identify your service needs

• Stage 4: Make and carry out a learning and action plan

• Stage 5: Document your learning, competence, performance and standards of service delivery

References

1   Chambers R, Wakley G, Field S and Ellis S (2003) *Appraisal for the Apprehensive*. Radcliffe Medical Press, Oxford.

2   Chambers R, Mohanna K, Wakley G and Wall D (2004) *Demonstrating Your Competence 1: healthcare teaching*. Radcliffe Medical Press, Oxford.

3   Eraut M and du Boulay B (2000) *Developing the Attributes of Medical Professional Judgement and Competence*. University of Sussex, Brighton. Reproduced at www.informatics.sussex. ac.uk/users/bend/doh

4   European Mentoring and Coaching Council (2004) *Code of Ethics*. European Mentoring and Coaching Council, Sherwood House, 7 Oxhey Road, Watford, Hertfordshire WD19 4QF or www.emccouncil.org

6

Helping the mentee to reach their potential

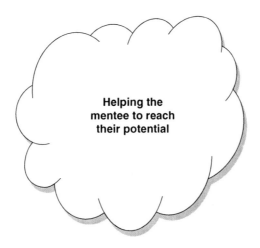

Helping the
mentee to reach
their potential

The tools and techniques described in this chapter will help you as a mentee to make the most of your mentoring sessions and the developmental opportunities that will emerge as you reflect on your current situation and make plans for the future. Many of the sections and activities directed at mentors in Chapter 3 can be generalised to mentees to a great extent, and you may wish to read and reflect on those tools and techniques as well.

The approaches in this chapter are suggestions that you might pick and choose from. Discuss with your mentor what activities might suit you and help your self-awareness or confidence levels. Then have a go ... reflect ... and change your practice or usual habits.

Karpman triangle[1]

The Karpman triangle illustrated in Figure 6.1 demonstrates at each point the personal and professional roles that you can play in your daily life.

- The persecutor.
- The victim.
- The rescuer.

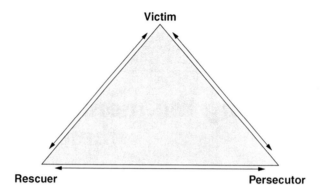

Figure 6.1:   The Karpman triangle.[1]

As situations change, so roles change. If a person in the triangle changes roles, this has implications for others changing their roles. The switching between these roles provides the 'drama'.

The *victim* 'Poor Me':

- feels victimised, oppressed, helpless, hopeless, powerless, ashamed
- looks for a rescuer who will perpetuate their negative feelings
- blocks themself from making decisions, solving problems, pleasure and self-understanding, if they stay in the victim position
- adopts a 'dejected' stance.

The *rescuer* with their 'Let me help you' approach:

- rescues when really they do not want to
- feels guilty if they do not rescue someone
- keeps victims dependent
- gives permission to others to fail
- expects to fail in rescue attempts.

The *persecutor* with their 'It's all your fault':

- sets strict limits unnecessarily
- blames
- criticises
- keeps victims oppressed
- is mobilised by anger
- adopts a rigid, authoritative stance
- acts as a 'critical parent'.

Activity 6.1: Think of a recent situation at work where you interacted with other colleagues. Picture yourself in one of the roles above throughout the 'drama' of the unfolding situation as you recall it.

• Where were you in the triangle throughout the 'drama'?

• What was the impact of the roles you played?

• What was the final outcome of the situation?

• What strategies might you use to help guide you in a more positive direction more quickly in future?

Be your own hero[2]

This tool could help you as a mentee to realise that being who you would like to be is possible. The exercise is a chance for people to rehearse their undeveloped ability and fulfil their potential. The mentor and mentee will need to do this exercise together.

Activity 6.2

1   Who is your hero? They may be real, fictional, dead or alive. You may want to draw them, or draw things you admire about them. What are the specific qualities you admire?

2   Imagine how your hero might behave on a very simple level, for example how might they walk around a room. Take on the persona of your hero and imagine a chat with somebody. What would your hero say and how would they behave? What advice might they give to others?

continued opposite

---

3 Next, think of a scenario from the past that did not go as well as you would have liked. This could be a problem you have experienced at work or at home; an interaction with another person; a struggle with learning or motivation or anything else that you can think of. Working with your mentor, play out the scenario as you remember it happening, including the negative outcome.

4 What would you have liked to have done differently? Re-enact the situation, but this time as your hero instead of your 'old self', in a more positive way. Try not to take action which is too fantastic. Focus instead on the superior, human qualities that your character has, and let them dictate your reactions.

5 Was the outcome positive this time? If so, how did it feel? How did you cope as your hero? Did you enjoy the feeling of release as well as success? Then ask yourself whether you were just acting as your hero or if you were uncovering hidden attributes in your own personality. It might well have felt strange, but this is because you are not used to behaving in this way. As with anything, practice makes perfect, so if this exercise was good for you then carry on assuming the qualities that you would like to have. In time, you will see that making a change is not so difficult, and that by acting as our heroes we can become more like them.

The rucksack exercise[2]

The purpose of this exercise is to help you to realise that you do not have to carry unnecessary 'baggage' around with you – it is easier to move around without it. This exercise can be imaginary, sitting inside a room with your mentor, or it can be liberating to undertake the exercise carrying the loaded rucksack itself. Both the mentee and mentor can arrange a walk (up a hill, around a park), taking with them a rucksack full of real rocks, each symbolising an experience that you would feel a greater sense of health and wellbeing if you were not carrying them around with you on a day-to-day basis.

Activity 6.3: Imagine you have a rucksack on your back. Every significant experience you have had in your life, whether good or bad, is represented by an imaginary rock that weighs the same as a large bag of sugar. You need to imagine a rock being dropped into your imaginary rucksack for every experience you have had.

As a guide, your life so far could be something like the following.

- You were born – experience.
- You have your first memory of food – experience.
- You learn to ride a bike – experience.
- You start school – experience.
- You discover maths – experience.
- You go through puberty – experience.
- You take exams – experience, experience ....

Carry on along these lines up to the present day, remembering to put a rock in your sack for every significant life event.

- How heavy is your rucksack once you have got to the present day?
- What does it feel like if you take off your rucksack? Lighter, easier, liberating?
- So why, then, do you think you have to carry this rucksack around with you the whole time?
- You have a choice. When you get out of bed in the morning do you put on your rucksack or simply head out into the world thinking what today might bring? It is clear that your life would be better if you did the latter. Your future depends on what action you are taking now, not what you did, or did not do, in the past.

The anchor experience[3]

Every one of us has felt as if we ruled the world at some point in our lives. It can be possible to tap into that feeling if you want to.

Activity 6.4

- Remember a moment when you were supremely confident. It does not matter when or where you were or what you were doing

- Once you have got the sensation of confidence then close your eyes and start to let that feeling increase. Now picture where you would like to carry this confidence with you. It may be to a party, a public-speaking event, playing sport, a job interview or just everyday living

- Picture yourself wherever you want to take your feeling of confidence – whether it is in an interview room or in front of an audience. Then start to increase that feeling of confidence even more

- Physically feel where the sensation of confidence is coming from. Is it from your stomach, your hands, your heart? Now start to throw this sensation around your body, running from your head to your feet and back up again. Increase the feeling even more. You may want to start counting from one to ten, raising the feeling of confidence in your body with each number

- Now that you are overflowing with confidence and about to explode, what do you do? What you need to do is think of an 'anchor'. The anchor is a physical gesture – anything from punching the air to giving your thigh a pinch. You should perform this anchor when you are at the point of 'maximum confidence'

- Follow this process a few times to get the hang of it as well as to make it more effective. What it will enable you to do is trigger off that feeling of confidence whenever you want. So if you are going into an interview and need a boost of confidence it could simply be a case of pinching your thigh and in you go, ready to conquer the world.

The three brains

* Your brain does the analytical thinking.
* Your gut reaction tells you if you are on the right track.
* Your heart confirms that you have done the right thing at the right time.

This exercise has also been adapted from BBC Health.[4]

Activity 6.5

* Ask the mentee to write the headings on a flip chart/sheet of paper and brainstorm each section considering all aspects of the issue from that angle. The mentor facilitates this thinking by using open questioning
* Draw mind maps from each of the brains: the mentor assists the mentee to explore the issues under each section and gives feedback about their body language when they were in each brain mode, indicating a preference or difficulty

---

Learning styles

Everyone has their preferred learning style(s). This means that there may be a mismatch between the preferred styles of the teacher and those they are addressing. So it is important that teachers are aware of their own preferences and how these might enrapture or bore people with other learning styles. The activities and learning techniques in this book should enable mentors to vary their styles and the mode of delivery to a particular mentee or between mentees.

Honey and Mumford have described four learning styles.[5–7]

* **Activists**: like to be fully involved in new experiences, open-minded, will try anything once, thrive on the challenge of new experiences but soon get bored and want to go on to the next challenge. They are gregarious and like to be the centre of attention. Activists learn best through new experiences, short activities, situations where they can be centre stage (chairing meetings, leading discussions), and when allowed to generate new ideas and have a go at things or brainstorm ideas.
* **Reflectors**: like to stand back, think about things thoroughly and collect a lot of information before coming to a conclusion. They are cautious, take a back seat in meetings and discussions, adopt a low profile, and appear tolerant and unruffled. When they do act it is by using the wide picture of their own and others' views. Reflectors learn best from situations where they are allowed to watch and think about activities before acting. They carry out research first, review the evidence, produce carefully constructed reports and can reach decisions in their own time.
* **Theorists**: like to adapt and integrate observations into logical maps and models, using step-by-step processes. They tend to be perfectionists, detached, analytical and objective. They reject anything that is subjective, flippant and lateral thinking in nature. Theorists learn best from activities where there are plans, maps and models to describe what is going on. When they are offered complex situations to understand and are intellectually stretched, they prefer to take time to explore the methodology and work with structured situations with a clear purpose.

- **Pragmatists**: like to try out ideas, theories and techniques to see if they work in practice. They will act quickly and confidently on ideas that attract them and are impatient with ruminating and open-ended discussions. They are down-to-earth people who like solving problems and making practical decisions, responding to problems as a challenge. Pragmatists learn best when there is an obvious link between the subject and their jobs. They enjoy trying out techniques with coaching and feedback, practical issues, real problems to solve and when they are given the immediate chance to implement what has been learned.

Convergent and divergent thinkers: there are several models describing learning styles that can be useful when designing learning opportunities. Convergent thinkers tend to find just one solution to a problem, but discussion and training can allow people to learn more divergent thinking skills, where new ideas and exploration of ideas is preferred. Divergent thinking is more useful in the real world where there are multiple opportunities.

Serialists learn one step after another and **holistic thinkers** prefer to look at the whole picture first and then focus in on the constituent parts. It is useful to think of this type of model when designing materials that will be used for self-development, as the material will need to suit both types of thinkers.

Activity 6.6

To self-assess your learning style you should complete the 80-item Learning Styles questionnaire[6] or attend a course where rating your learning style is an integral part of the programme.

Time management[8]

Better time management is often a skill that mentees prioritise after discussion with their mentor. The many ways to manage your time better fall into three main categories.

1 **Reducing the amount of work to be done** by refusing it in the first place, delegating it, or doing less of it.
2 **Doing the work more quickly** by doing it less thoroughly or processing it more efficiently.
3 **Allowing more time for the particular piece of work** so that there is less time pressure on completing it.

Prioritise your time – do not allow yourself or others to waste it. The first step is to be clear about your goals in your work and home lives, or leisure. Then you need to structure sufficient time around those priorities. When an activity arises over which you have choice, match it against your goals. If it takes you further away from your goals, then refuse to take it on, but if it coincides with your goals, consider if you have time to fit it in.

Make sure you spend your quality time doing the most important or complex jobs. It is too easy to focus on getting small, unimportant tasks done and put off tackling the big ones, which just hang over you and make you feel guilty for leaving them un-attended. A high-priority task has to be done, a medium-priority job may be delegated and a low-priority task should only be done if you have no medium- or high-priority tasks waiting, or you are too jaded to tackle them. The majority of your time should be devoted to pursuing your most important goals, and a small proportion of your time spent on less-important matters.

Control interruptions – interruptions are one of the biggest timewasters, especially if someone else could have handled the problem or taken the message or no action was required. Even if an interruption is necessary, it may occur at the wrong time, wrecking your concentration or train of thought. Agree rules in your workplace for who may be interrupted and when.

Include sufficient time for thinking, doing, meeting, developing and learning. You need to be fresh and creative to stay on top of the demands made on you. You can only manage this in the longer term if you have the right mix of stimulating work, personal and professional development, and networking regularly timetabled into your daily schedule. You will achieve more in designated sessions of quiet, uninterrupted periods than in a longer allotment of time broken up by various activities. You need uninter-rupted time for concentrating on planning, writing reports or analysing progress.

Try to allow at least 10% of your time for dealing with unexpected tasks. In the unlikely event that everything goes smoothly and you do not need the extra time, it will be a bonus to have that additional space to catch up on the backlog of paperwork, or simply spend a little more time talking to people about how they are feeling or what they are doing.

Delegate whatever and however you can – only accept delegated work if you have the necessary skills, time and experience. If you are in a position to delegate work and responsibilities, decide what only *you* can do and delegate as much as possible of the rest to others. If you are more usually on the receiving end of delegated work, try to make sure you understand what is required and that you have the necessary time, skills and experience before agreeing or acquiescing to taking on new work. If you do not have the time or skills for the additional work, negotiate in your most assertive manner how you will get the training and when you will do the work.

Do not just consider delegation at work, but at home too – cleaning, gardening, help from all the family with the chores, etc.

Control your work flow – concentrate on one task at a time. Complete it and either move on to another job or take a short break to refresh yourself and clear your mind ready to start again. Do not move from one task to another or you will waste effort, having to start thinking about the topic all over again each time you take it up.

You are likely to be more efficient if you group small, similar tasks together, such as returning phonecalls. Always have one or two small jobs put by or carried with you, so that if you are kept waiting you can get on with those jobs and not waste time. Maintain control of your paperwork. Do not let it build up so that you feel overwhelmed, or you will put off tackling it at all or work more slowly as the enormity of the task depresses you.

Limit the time you spend on the telephone. If you measure how long you talk for the next few times you are on the phone, you will probably be surprised by how many minutes the calls last.

Minimise paperwork – only pick up a piece of paper once, only start a job when you have time to finish it, deal with the most complicated task first while you are fresh, delegate appropriately as far as possible. Sort paperwork into:

- must be done today
- can wait a few days
- can wait a few weeks
- for someone else to do.

Activity 6.7: Keep a log of daily activities

Photocopy the daily log overleaf. Record your activities each day for a week, including off-duty time. Sort the activities into three separate columns:

- *personal needs*, including shopping, sleeping, domestic chores, bodily needs, etc.
- *work*, including reading work-related books, reports and papers
- *leisure*, including sport, relaxation, reading, music, etc.

Once you have worked out totals for the types of activity for each day, you should group the activities within the categories: personal needs, work and leisure. Compare several days of daily recordings for these categories with the Health Education Authority's (now the Health Development Agency) recommendations for a healthy lifestyle:

- 45–55% on personal needs
- 25–30% on work
- 20–25% on leisure.

Look for any trends or patterns of activities – such as staying late at work or catching up on paperwork at home. Do you think you can improve the way you divide your own time? Could you change the extent to which you have a good balance in the way you allocate time to essential, desirable and unimportant activities in your life? Discuss your log with your partner or family at home or a work colleague.

Daily log of activities

Time spent (to nearest quarter of an hour) on

Personal needs (shopping, washing, domestic chores, sleeping)		Work		Leisure	
Activity	*Time spent*	*Activity*	*Time spent*	*Activity*	*Time spent*
Total/day		*Total/day*		*Total/day*	

Activity 6.8: Reduce time pressures at work[8,9]

Use this activity to look at the suggestions for reducing time pressures that are listed below from the perspectives of an individual and an organisation

What you can do as an individual	*What the organisation can do*
Plan well in advance to avoid crises	Plan well in advance to avoid crises
Allow 10% of your time for unexpected tasks	Organise time management training for staff
Do not book a meeting too close to a previous commitment that may overrun	Match staff numbers to volume of work
Build in time for reflection and planning	Organise realistic work plans
Minimise interruptions	Discourage social chitchat in work time
Make maximum use of technology	Make maximum use of technology
Other:	Other:

Action points to reduce time pressures
What you will do:

As an individual	*And when*	*As an organisation*	*And when*
1			
2			
3			
4			
5			

Undertaking this activity will force you to realise the varied solutions available for reducing time pressures and that you are not helpless. It will also help you as a mentee to understand that you cannot reduce time pressures on you as an individual in isolation from the rest of the organisation. Both the individual and organisation need to work together to reduce time pressures effectively.

Keeping a reflective learning log[8]

As a mentee working in the NHS you should have a permanent record of your learning to keep in your portfolio. Evidence of learning can be extracted at a later date if it is required for supervision, appraisal, revalidation or re-accreditation of your professional registration. It will be useful to review your portfolio, or the parts you are happy to make 'public,' with your mentor from time to time.

Activity 6.9: You can use your reflective learning log to pick out the most personally significant experiences on a particular day and record what you learned from the experience(s). This will involve reflecting on:

- what was most significant
- why this was personally significant
- what you learned
- any actions you propose to take as a result.

Do not restrict yourself to a particular event. You can also use the log to record other thoughts, ideas, insights and feelings. You might also record what worked for you and what did not, and the reasons. Other observations might include the relevance of the learning to your work or personal life. Using a reflective log in this way will help you to become more aware of how and what you are learning. Keeping a log reminds people who squeeze learning in between other activities they perceive as more important and rush off home or back to work, to spend time on reflection.

Stress management[8,9]

The types of practical method mentees and others can use to cope with stress at work include:

- seeking support from colleagues
- sharing problems with colleagues
- adopting better time-management practices
- more appropriate booking times for appointments and meetings
- increased protected time off-duty, limiting working hours to those for which you are contracted
- admitting doubts and worries to others
- achieving a better balance between work and home commitments.

Avoid being a workaholic and instead:

- stop being a perfectionist
- do not judge your mistakes too harshly
- resist the desire to control everything
- learn to decline extra commitments assertively if you are already pressed for time
- look after your personal health and fitness
- allow time for personal growth, the family and leisure
- do not be too proud to ask for help.

It is not stress itself that is the damaging factor but your inability to cope with it. In a changing world, people need to learn new ways of coping. That way lies survival. Only you can identify the best stress-managing solutions for you. It may help you to decide which stress-reducing interventions you want to make if you classify interventions as being:

- preventive, i.e. to reduce or change the nature of the stressor, to remove the 'hazard' or reduce the frequency/extent of the stressor
- altering your individual response to stress or improving your ability to recognise and deal with stress-related problems as they arise
- minimising the effects of stress, i.e. to heal/help those who have been traumatised or stressed by their work; obtain help so you can cope with and recover from problems at work.

Activity 6.10: Undertake your own significant event audit of stress from work

Analyse a significant event at work

- Stage 1: Write down a factual account of the stressful situation you have chosen – who was involved, the time of day and the task/activity you or others were doing

- Stage 2: Write down the reasons for the crisis or stressful situation arising from your specific situation

- Stage 3: Write down the effects of stress on you and the participants in the crisis or stressful situation you have chosen

continued overleaf

- Stage 4: Record how you or others might have behaved differently, or how the organisation might be changed to reduce or eliminate this cause of stress from occurring

Analyse the significant event with your mentor or colleagues at work, to draw out more insights and new ideas for solutions

---

Activity 6.11: Undertake your own significant event audit of stress from outside work

Analyse a significant event audit outside of work

- Stage 1: Write down a factual account of the stressful situation you have chosen – who was involved, the time of day and the task/activity you or others were doing

- Stage 2: Write down the reasons for the crisis or stressful situation arising from your specific situation

continued opposite

- Stage 3: Write down the effects of stress on you and the participants in the crisis or stressful situation you have chosen

- Stage 4: Record how you or others might have behaved differently, or how the workplace/home organisation might be changed to reduce or eliminate the cause of stress you have nominated from occurring

Analyse the significant event with your mentor or family and friends, to draw out more insights and new ideas for solutions

Be assertive[8]

Assertiveness is about knowing and practising your rights – to change your mind, to make mistakes, to refuse demands, to express emotions, to be yourself without having to act for other people's benefit, and to make decisions or statements without having always to justify them. It takes practice to be assertive – so get some practice in at work and at home. The biggest challenge may be being assertive with yourself so that you don't agree to take on additional tasks that are not essential for you to undertake, or that fall outside your own priority areas.

How often do you hear people saying: 'No, no ... no ... oh ... alright then, I suppose so'? Listen carefully to what is being asked of you, weigh up the time, effort and skills the task or activity will take, and the extent to which it is an essential, desirable or possible feature of your working or home lives – and decide on your assertive response.

There are 12 key points to remember about being assertive.

1   Say 'No' clearly and then move away or change the subject. Keep repeating 'No' – don't be diverted.
2   Be honest and direct with everyone.

3   Don't apologise or justify yourself more than is reasonable.
4   Offer a workable compromise and negotiate an agreement that suits you and the other party.
5   Pause before answering with a 'Yes' you will regret. Delay your response and give yourself more time to think by asking for more information.
6   Be aware of your body language and keep it as assertive as possible. Match your tone to your words (do not smile if you are giving a serious message).
7   Use the 'broken record' technique – persistently repeat your message in a calm manner to someone who is trying to pressurise you. Don't be side-tracked.
8   Show that you are listening to the other person's point of view and giving them a fair hearing.
9   Practise expressing your opinion and rights rather than expecting other people to guess what you want.
10 Do not be too hard on yourself if you make a mistake – everyone is human.
11 Be confident enough to change your mind if that is appropriate.
12 It can be assertive to say nothing.

Activity 6.12: Consider your usual body language when in situations where you disagree with others over an issue that you consider to be important.

Non-verbal behaviour: the body language that gives you away

Passive	Assertive	Aggressive
Covers mouth with hand	Direct eye contact	Gesticulates expansively
Looks down at the floor	Head erect	Clenched/pounding fists
Constant shifting of weight	Descriptive hand gestures	Finger pointing
Fiddles with clothing	Emphasises key words	Hands on hips
Rubs head or parts of body	Steady, firm voice	Rigid posture
Frequent nodding of head	Open movements	Strident voice
Throat clearing	Relaxed	Stares others down

Do you recognise your non-verbal behaviour patterns from the list above as mainly 'passive', mainly 'assertive', or mainly 'aggressive' in a:

• situation at work with a patient?
• situation at work with other colleagues?
• outside work with a shop assistant?
• outside work with a member of your family?

Are you consistent? Do you behave differently at work from how you do at home or in another setting? Could you change your non-verbal behaviour and the signals you give out so that you behave more consistently?

Seek support[8]

Research into stress has shown that people with the best social supports who interact well with other people are able to cope with stress and are the least affected by it. Be prepared to ask for help – it is not a sign of weakness or ignorance. Support networks may be used for another professional opinion or for emotional assistance. Support for colleagues should be non-judgemental and a culture developed at work where people do not feel embarrassed or silly to be asking for help. A close and supportive spouse and family at home can be a good, safe place to offload and share worries about work, so long as this does not stress relationships unduly.

Activity 6.13

Draw up a personal map of support mechanisms in your life. Undertaking this exercise will help you to realise for yourself the components of your life that lend you support, that you can build on.

- Stage 1: Draw yourself in the middle of a piece of plain paper. Then draw pictures to represent all the sources of support in your life – people, things, situations, environment, etc. Link each picture to you in the centre with a line (*see* the example on page 133)

- Stage 2: Next add in drawings of what other sources of support you have used in the past but not employed for a while, and add other pictures of what extra sources of support you would like to have. Link each picture to you in the centre of the page

- Stage 3: Draw in the barriers that stop you using these sources of support across the line linking that particular source with you

- Stage 4: Share and compare your personal support map with your mentor or someone else who has drawn one. Discuss which are your strongest sources of support, which are the ones you would like to enhance, the presence of the barriers that stop you making more of your sources of support and what is missing

It will help you to acknowledge and review the extent and type of the sources of support that exist for you at work or outside work. Have some previous sources of support withered away? Are you taking your partner or family for granted and not devoting enough quality time to them? Can you recognise the barriers that stop you from spending time and effort on leisure activities or maintaining your interpersonal relationships at work or home?

continued overleaf

Make a plan to remove at least one barrier to enhance at least one source of support.

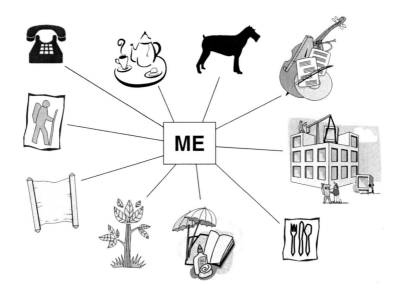

Figure 6.2:   Example of a personal support map (reproduced from Schwartz[9]).

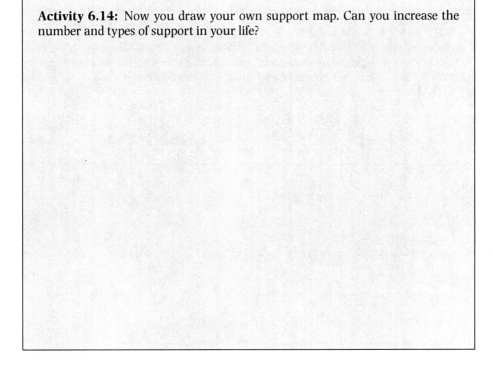

Activity 6.14: Now you draw your own support map. Can you increase the number and types of support in your life?

Raise your self-esteem[9,10]

Even confident-seeming people may suffer from low self-esteem. Some people blame the hierarchy in the NHS for their loss of self-esteem. You can deliberately raise your self-esteem by positive tactics and thinking, but to effect any change you have to be prepared to take the risk of failure – success is not automatic. And to ride failures successfully you have to develop a positive approach before you start, so that you can set yourself up to learn from failure rather than be cast down by it.

Ten positive strategies to raise your self-esteem.

1   Accept that not every attempt to change will be a success.
2   Be prepared to take a risk to effect a change in your life.
3   Try positive visualisation, that is imagine yourself successfully managing a forthcoming event or activity about which you are feeling apprehensive.
4   Use positive body language – people will treat you more positively too.
5   Review and recall past successes and hold them in the forefront of your mind.
6   Learn from any mistakes or failures and do not dismiss such experiences.
7   Learn to feel comfortable with yourself – physically and mentally.
8   Write your worries down and review them periodically rather than continually fretting over them.
9   Be aware of your good points and constantly reinforce them in your thinking.
10 Do the best for yourself and give yourself every opportunity to succeed – do not set yourself up to fail.

Activity 6.15: Review the state of your self-esteem. Do you need to concentrate on trying to raise your self-esteem? If so, write down any positive strategies you could take to raise your self-esteem; if your self-esteem is pretty good what can you do to maintain it? What will you do and when?

1

2

3

4

Make a plan to review the outcomes of this exercise

Making changes in your life

Change can be an emotionally and physically stressful time in your life. In today's climate, there are constant changes and challenges facing you, often from more than one source at a time, e.g. from your family, clients, colleagues and managers. It is therefore vital to learn to deal with these at every level. Before you can influence or change other aspects of your life, you need to learn how to manage yourself. This in turn will have a profound effect in withstanding other external forces.

Activity 6.16: Consider the following questions and statements which are outlined under the five themes below and develop an action plan to help enhance your change agent skills and abilities.

Learning to manage yourself   **Actions**

- What are your strengths for
  implementing change?

- What are your development needs?

- How receptive are you to new ideas
  and innovations?

- How do you respond to people who
  are not as committed to the change
  process as you feel they should be?

- How do you respond to criticism of
  any new ideas that you may have?

**Building, developing and maintaining
effective relationships**

- Have you identified who needs to be
  involved and communicated with
  about this change?

continued overleaf

- Plan your communication strategy.
  How effective are your communication
  skills?

- Think about people who are external
  to your immediate team, other disciplines,
  departments and the wider organisation.
  How effective are your links to these people
  and within the wider organisation?

- How receptive are you to new ideas and
  innovations generated by team members?

- What are your strengths in terms of
  influencing other people?

Patient/client focus

- Have the patients/clients requested/
  identified this change?

- If not, have they been consulted about
  this change? What are their thoughts?

- How will this change improve patient care?

- Will the change add value to patient care?

- How will the implementation of this change
  benefit the service you deliver to
  patients/clients?

continued opposite

Political awareness

- Are you loyal, open and honest about the change process?

- Can you deal effectively with criticism and with being disliked?

- Are you aware of the personal impact that changes may have on individuals?

- Are you tactful and emotionally intelligent?

- Do you check information and rumour?

- Can you build effective alliances?

- Do you know who can and who cares?

- Are you skilled at negotiating and listening?

Networking

- Has this change being implemented elsewhere (within or external to the organisation, locally, nationally or internationally)?

- If so, what can you learn from the experience of others?

continued overleaf

- How can you best share good practice (within or external to the organisation, locally, nationally or internationally)?

- How good are your systems to share good practice and learn from others?

References

1 Karpman S (1968) Fairy tales and script drama analysis. *Transactional Analysis Bulletin 7.* **26**: 39–43.

2 Leighton R (2002) *Confidence Lab. Improving Lives in 7 Days.* BBC Health, London.

3 Cohen P (2002) *Confidence Lab. Improving Lives in 7 Days.* BBC Health, London.

4 Cooper C (2002) *Confidence Lab. Improving Lives in 7 Days.* BBC Health, London.

5 Honey P and Mumford A (1986) *Using Your Learning Styles.* Peter Honey, Maidenhead.

6 Honey P and Mumford A (2000) *The Learning Styles Questionnaire 80-Item Version.* Peter Honey, Maidenhead.

7 Mohanna K, Wall D and Chambers R (2004) *Teaching Made Easy. A Manual for Health Professionals* (2e). Radcliffe Medical Press, Oxford.

8 Chambers R (1999) *Survival Skills for GPs.* Radcliffe Medical Press, Oxford.

9 Chambers R, Schwartz A and Boath E (2003) *Beating Stress in the NHS.* Radcliffe Medical Press, Oxford.

10 Chambers R, Wakley G, Iqbal Z and Field S (2002) *Prescription for Learning. Techniques, Games and Activities.* Radcliffe Medical Press, Oxford.

7

Documentation

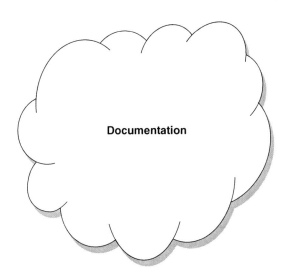

Documentation

Template for a job description and person specification of a mentor based on the NHS Knowledge and Skills Framework

1 General details

	Organisation's name:
Job title:	Mentor
Location:	Base, e.g. trust
Time commitment:	Minimum of A mentoring sessions lasting minimum of B hours per mentee, within 12-month period
Names of mentees:	XX, YY (maximum numbers of mentees is ... minimum is one)
Contract status:	Options: Volunteer/Self-employed/Employed as part of normal job role, etc.
Additional allowances:	Sessional fee (if relevant); travel, training, etc. payable
Tenure:	Accreditation by (trust, college, deanery?) every 3 years
Accountable to:	Mentoring lead

2 Main purpose

To act as a mentor to one or more individuals in accordance with the definition of mentoring: a 'process whereby the mentor guides the mentee in the development and re-examination of their own ideas, learning, and personal and professional development' (Standing Committee on Postgraduate Medical and Dental Education (SCOPME) (1998) *Supporting Doctors and Dentists at Work. An Enquiry into Mentoring.* SCOPME, London).

3 Declaration

The mentor must declare at selection and re-selection (and if pertinent, while in post) that he/she is not currently under investigation for any criminal offence or General Medical Council (GMC)/Nursing and Midwifery Council (NMC)/Health Professions Council (HPC)/local procedure, which might bring the mentoring process into disrepute.

4 Core competencies

Mentors are expected to take an active part in their own development and that of their mentees, as well as other peers in participating in mentoring scheme activities locally and at the organisational level (e.g. trust, deanery).

- **Communication skills:** consistently practise good communication skills with mentees and organisation (e.g. trust), recognise and take account of the mentee's favoured interpersonal style in order to optimise communication, establish rapport, use active listening, summarise, negotiate and give constructive feedback. Recognise and sensitively manage areas of resistance and conflict within the discussion process and be able to challenge the belief constructively.
- **Personal and people development:** develop own and others' knowledge and practice across professional and organisational boundaries in relation to mentoring. Understand the healthcare context relevant to the mentee and make realistic allowances for problems and issues (including the mentee's attitudes, beliefs, learning style, motivation, etc.) that might obstruct the application of best practice. Talk and respond knowledgeably about the competing demands within the mentor's everyday work, while understanding national and local healthcare priorities and how these are relevant to the mentee's circumstances.
- **Health and safety and risk management:** promote others' health, safety and security in relation to mentoring; have network for referral, e.g. occupational health, help for stress, financial or relationship difficulties, both within and outside the NHS.
- **Service development: develop and improve NHS services through mentoring:** encourage reflective practice to enable the mentee to learn from his/her own experience. Be able to recognise and acknowledge whether learning has occurred since the previous meeting and whether it has addressed the mentee's needs.
- **Quality improvement:** demonstrate personal commitment to quality improvement, offering others advice and support as integral part of mentoring.
- **Equality, diversity and rights:** enable others to exercise their rights, and promote equal opportunities and diversity through mentoring. Be aware of *own* values, beliefs and attitudes, and seek to use these in a constructive manner, principally, but not exclusively, in the interests of the mentee. Make evaluations and provide feedback that is free of bias and prejudice, be open and transparent in dealings involving the mentee and maintain confidentiality unless required by duty or statute to do otherwise.

- **Promotion of self-care and peer support:** encourage others to promote their own current and future health and wellbeing, through mentoring. Be sensitive to mentee's health concerns that may impair performance and/or judgement.
- **Partnership and support:** develop and sustain partnership working with mentees and organisation (e.g. trust or deanery). Attempt to understand and resolve disputes. Have good influencing skills – seeking information, testing understanding, labelling behaviour and commentating on feelings. Foster good working relationships with other parts of the health service.
- **Leadership skills:** lead others in the development of knowledge, ideas and work practice as an integral part of mentoring. Recognise own leadership skills and those of others. Be able to develop leadership in others. Recognise qualities in the mentee that the mentee wants to develop. Support the mentee in developing his/ her values and in working in an ethical professional framework and help mentee to develop his/her professional skills and personal attributes.
- **Protected time:** identify and negotiate protected time to devote to mentoring process, and take active part in local learning sets for peer support (if appropriate).

Date job description revised June 2004
Variation to job description
The XX organisation reserves the right to vary the duties and responsibilities of its employees or those with whom they are contracting to provide mentoring services, within the general conditions of the Scheme of pay and conditions and related matters. Thus it must be appreciated that the duties and responsibilities outlined above may be altered as the changing needs of the service may require.

Person specification assessment form for mentor

Candidate: Trust:

Post title: Mentor   Date:

Essential (E) and Desirable (D) factors for post *Please tick as appropriate*			*Assessment/notes*
A Education	E	D	
Health-related degree/qualification		✔	
Satisfactory completion of mentor training	✔		
B Experience			
Work as XX (health) currently or within previous two years	✔		
Background in training and development		✔	
C Specific skills, aptitudes and knowledge	E	D	
Experience of life		✔	
Communication skills	✔		
Development of personal and people development	✔		
Health and safety and risk management	✔		
Knowledge and skills relating to mentoring	✔		
Quality improvement	✔		
Equal opportunities and diversity	✔		
Leadership skills	✔		
Up-to-date clinical skills	✔		
Well versed in NHS context		✔	
Counselling skills		✔	
D Personal qualities			
Has self-confidence	✔		
Be intuitive	✔		
E Can create protected time for mentoring	✔		
F Health/physical abilities			
Physically and psychologically capable of undertaking the work as a mentor	✔		

Overall assessment/General comment

Completed by:

Mentee application form

Surname: First name:

Current post:

Preferred contact address:

Contact numbers: 1

                            2

                            3

Best hours to contact me on above number:

Fax number:

Email address:

Work address:

Work contact numbers: 1

                            2

Best hours to contact me on above number:

Today's date: ....

Please return this form to:
Administrator
[postal address /email]

Mentor application form

In preparation for the mentor training, we would like you to consider the programme and its application to you as a person fully. In order to be considered for the programme, would you please fill in and return this confidential application form. By its very nature, the work of mentoring is individual and relies on a mentor's understanding and awareness of working with other people as well as their personal insight.

Name: Occupation:

How long have you been working in this profession?

Write a short paragraph outlining why you are interested in becoming a mentor.

How would you describe yourself? Write a brief summary:

What skills, experience and interests do you have that you feel would help you to be a good mentor?
What do you hope to gain from mentor training?

Prompts:

- Demonstrable personal and professional development track record
- Evidence of sharing learning with others
- Respected as an honest, trustworthy individual
- Approachable and discreet
- Understand the environment, current climate and NHS changes
- Willing and able to commit time and energy to the mentoring contract
- Up-to-date skills, expertise and knowledge

Reproduced with permission of 4 Health Ltd.

Please give the names of two referees who would be willing to comment on your suitability as a mentor.

Reproduced with permission: Schwartz & Brisby/Arcadia Alive Ltd, Arcadia Alive, Human Factors Consultancy, Parkfield Centre, Park Street, Stafford ST17 4AL

Mentor initial training programme – an example

Reproduced with permission of Schwartz & Brisby/Arcadia Alive Ltd., Arcadia Alive, Human Factors Consultancy, Parkfield Centre, Park Street, Stafford ST17 4AL.

Objectives

By the end of the course participants will:

- understand the meaning of mentoring and how it differs from other forms of support and training
- have learnt and practised the essential skills of acting as a mentor
- have explored methods of working to reduce stress and promote constructive change
- have a clear understanding of the ethical basis for mentoring
- recognise the need for ongoing quality control of mentoring, and accept means of ensuring that in relation to their own practice.

Participants and quality of learning/training

Taking into account the experiential nature of the training in mentoring skills (including coaching, listening and facilitation skills), and the need for close supervision during the training, the ideal number of participants is between eight and 12.

Outline programme

Best practice would be to run this programme over at least two days, but if time is limited, it may be condensed to 1.5 days.

Day one

Approximate times	Session content	Style, presentation, equipment
9.30–10.00	Introductions Expectations of the course Ground rules Ice-breakers: • leaving baggage behind • mindfulness exercise	Group discussion Input
10.00–10.30	What is mentoring? Why is it important? Making a case for it – what use is mentoring? What are the skills required? Experiences of mentoring and coaching Mentoring style and communication	Group discussion Flip chart
10.30–11.00	How mentoring differs from: support, coaching, counselling, training Roles and responsibilities of mentor/mentee. Building the relationship – developing rapport Establishing a contract for mentoring Developing the mentee. Disabling qualities	Input PowerPoint Group discussion
11.00–11.15	Coffee	
11.15–12.00	Mentoring is about change! The framework: • personal • professional • strategic • operational How do people make changes? Experiential exercise: a period of change...	Input PowerPoint Exercise in pairs
12.00–12.30	Feedback on the exercise Are there secondary gains from staying 'stuck'? What about the 'learned helplessness' syndrome? What about staying with the 'messy bit'?	Group discussion
12.30–1.00	Model of development, change and loss	Input

continued opposite

Approximate times	Session content	Style, presentation, equipment
1.00–1.45	Lunch – time for networking and noticing using mindfulness approach	
1.45–2.45	Refer back to session before lunch: what helped you to be able to make the necessary changes?	Group
2.45–3.00	Input on basic skills of listening, coaching and facilitation Exploration – understanding – action	Input plus handouts
3.00–3.45	Skills practice – using case scenarios – on the exploration stage: • active listening • paraphrasing • open questions • use of silence	Group work Pairs/threes
3.45–4.00	Tea	
4.00–4.30	Feedback on the exercises Review of the day Plans for day two	Group discussion Input

Day two (consisting of one half-day)

Approximate times	Session content	Style, presentation, equipment
9.30–9.45	Exercise to refocus on the tasks: • leaving baggage behind	Group exercise
9.45–10.00	Personal constructs and mentoring Relevance to mentoring: choice of and characteristics of a mentor	Input
10.00–10.30	Input on basic and advanced skills *Basic skills* Active listening, paraphrasing, summarising and open questions *Advanced skills* Challenging, taking a strategic perspective, focusing forward, developing an action plan	Input plus handouts
10.30–11.15	Skills practice – using scenario	Pairs/threes
11.15–11.30	Coffee	

continued overleaf

Approximate times	Session content	Style, presentation, equipment
11.30–12.00	Application of mentoring: planning tool The role of mentors How to move this forward	Input PowerPoint Handout Exercise
12.00–12.15	Mentoring, coaching, listening Why are we doing this then? Practical and ethical issues Support and quality control • confidentiality • note taking • boundaries • limits of competence • onward referrals • supervision and ongoing training	Group exercise Group discussion Flip chart Linked with previous exercise
12.15–12.45	Summary What about support? Mapping it!	Group exercise
12.45–13.00	Feedback Review of the two days Close	Group discussion

Ongoing training and supervision

There should be a follow-up half-day after participants have had some experience, and the content of this day should include further skills practice plus consideration of any issues that have arisen. During this period mentors should be able to reflect and evaluate their mentoring as well as their mentee's progress.

Approximate times	Session content	Style, presentation, equipment
9.30–10.00	Introduction Expectations of the review session	Group discussion Input
10.00–10.45	What have we learnt about mentoring? Experiences Opportunities to reflect Positives, negatives, concerns Boundaries, referral on ...	Group discussion Flip chart
10.45–11.00	Advanced skills	Input PowerPoint Group discussion
11.00–11.15	Coffee	
11.15–12.00	Mentoring questions How to encourage creativity? Maintaining the relationship What are the blocks, patterns, personal challenges?	Input PowerPoint Exercise in pairs
12.00–12.30	Ongoing supervision and support Establishing support groups/buddies Ongoing learning	Group discussion
12.30–1.00	Feedback Evaluation Close	Group discussion Questionnaires

Mentee initial training programme – an example

2.00pm	Welcome, introductions and overview of the mentoring scheme
2.30pm	Commitment to the process: roles and responsibilities of mentors and mentees
3.00pm	Clarifying the mentoring relationship, establishing boundaries
3.30pm	Coffee taken during discussion around role of mentors
4.00pm	Introduction to the mentoring contract: defining personal learning outcomes
4.45pm	Productive behaviours for mentoring relationships: giving and receiving feedback, challenging perceptions and reflective practice
5.45pm	Selecting a mentor – discussion
6.00pm	Plenary

Reproduced with permission of 4 Health Ltd.

Mentoring confidentiality policy

1 Mentors are bound by a duty of confidentiality. This is a duty not to reveal any information disclosed to any third party.
2 This duty is applicable irrespective of the position in the organisation of the mentor or mentee.
3 The only exemption to the duty of the mentor's confidentiality will apply in respect of any information disclosed by the mentee relating to any illegal act or threat to patient safety. In the event of such a situation the mentor must tell the mentee at the time of discussion that they are unable to maintain confidentiality.
4 The commitment to confidentiality continues after the mentor and mentee have concluded their mentoring contract.
5 It is the responsibility of the mentee to keep any records/action plans up to date and in a safe place.

Signatures

Mentee: _____ Mentor: _____

NB A copy of this should be held by both parties.

Report after first mentoring session

Private and confidential
Please tick relevant box:

☐   I wish to continue mentoring sessions with my assigned mentor:

  ....

☐   I do not wish to continue mentoring sessions.
    Please give brief details:

  ....

  ....

  ....

☐   I wish to continue mentoring sessions with a change of mentor.

Mentee signature: ....

Print name: ....

At the end of your first meeting with your mentor please complete and return to:
Scheme administrator
[postal address]
Email:
Fax:

Mentoring contract

Parties involved:

- Mentor: ....
- Mentee: ....

Duration of mentoring arrangement: 6 months   1 year   18 months

Meeting frequency:

Meeting duration:

Expectations of the mentor by the mentee:

-
-
-
-
-
-

Expectations of the mentee by the mentor:

-
-
-
-
-

Each session should be preceded with a planning sheet outlining the topics to be discussed, issues the mentee wishes to raise and feedback from the last session.

This information can be emailed or faxed to the mentor no later than the day before the meeting, but preferably a couple of days' notice allows for preparation.

Signed: .... Mentor

Signed: .... Mentee

NB A copy of this document should be held by both parties.

Reproduced with permission of 4 Health Ltd.

Personal record of mentoring meetings

(Photocopy one for each meeting)

Mentee: Mentor:
Name: Name:
Place: Place:
Date: Place:

Mentoring prompt list (reproduced with kind permission of 4 Health Ltd)

What has happened since the last meeting?
- Update on learning; shifts, wins and insights.
- New situations/issues that need dealing with?
- New choices or decisions made?

What I am currently working on
- Progress report on goals, problems and activities.
- What are you proud of that you have achieved?
- What barriers are you coming up against?

Can my mentor help?
- Where am I stuck?
- A plan of action.
- A strategy or mechanism.

Next?
- What is the next learning outcome/development area you wish to tackle?
- What do you want for yourself next?

Record of meeting: agenda items planned
1
2
3
4
5

Reflections
What was discussed?

What did I feel?

Mentoring meetings action plan
(Please photocopy one for each meeting)

Areas identified	Actions to be taken	Resources available	By when?

Keep your actions SMART: (**S**pecific, **M**easurable, **A**chievable, **R**ealistic and **T**ime-scaled)

Date/Time/Place of next meeting:

Learning diary sheet

A learning diary can help to identify what is being learnt and how it is being transferred into practice.

- Record the learning that has taken place to be clear about the facts.
- Record feelings, reactions and judgements about the learning.
- Assess the relevance and application of the learning.

What did I do and how did I do it?

What was the significant learning?

Conclusions/learning points

Reaction to the learning

Action plan – how will I apply the learning?

Log record sheet of mentoring meetings

Name: _____

Mentor: _____

Session	Date	Duration	Next session	Mentor's signature	Mentee's signature
One					
Two					
Three					
Four					
Five					
Six					
Seven					
Eight					
Nine					
Ten					

Further reading

Alfred G, Garvey B and Smith R (2000) *The Mentoring Pocket Book.* Management Pocket Books, Hants.

Brooks V and Sikes P (1997) *The Good Mentor Guide.* Initial Teacher Education. Open University Press, Buckingham.

Butterworth T and Faugier J (1995) *Clinical Supervision and Mentorship in Nursing.* Chapman and Hall, London.

Clutterbuck D (2001) *Advances in Mentoring: ideas for the development of mentoring in the health context.* European Mentoring and Coaching Centre, Sheffield Hallam University, Sheffield.

Clutterbuck D (2001) *Everyone Needs a Mentor. How to Further Talent Within an Organisation.* Institute of Personnel Management, London.

Coldwell B and Carter EMA (1993) *The Return of the Mentor. Strategies for Workshop Learning.* Falmer Press, London.

Daloz LA (1986) *Effective Teaching and Mentoring: realising the transformational power of adult learning experiences.* Falmer Press, London.

Moreton-Cooper A and Palmer A (2000) *Mentoring, Perception and Clinical Supervision* (2e). Blackwell Science, London.

Parsloe E and Wray W (2000) *Coaching and Mentoring: practical methods to improve learning.* Kogan Page, London.

Royal College of Nursing (2001) *RCN Clinical Leadership Toolkit.* RCN, London.

Index

reflective learning log 126
reflective practice
  encouraging 12
  feelings 91
  guidelines 82
reflectors, learning style 120
relationships, building 51–2
reports, documentation 150
rescuers, Karpman triangle 113–15
resources
  mentoring schemes 19
  signposting 77
reviewing, mentoring relationship 33–4
rights 89–93
risk management 75–80
roles
  appraisers 9
  assessors 9
  clinical supervisors 9
  coaches 8–9
  counsellors 8
  mentors 17, 30–2
  preceptors 9
  supervisors 9
  teams 97
Royal College of Obstetricians and
      Gynaecologists (RCOG), mentoring
      schemes 23
rucksack exercise, baggage 118

safety/security/health 75–80, 93–6
schemes, mentoring see mentoring schemes
searching for mentors 14
security/health/safety 75–80, 93–6
self-care, promoting 93–6
self-development, enhancing 12
self-esteem
  raising 13
  see also confidence
self-management, mentees 28–9
serialists, learning style 121
service development 80–4
significant event auditing, quality
      improvement 87–9
skills 37–40
  communication see communication skills

competence 40
  KSF 38–40
  leadership 98–104
standard prodding, mentors' role 17
strengths analysis 83–4
stress 77
stress management 126–9
  see also support
success, encouraging 35
supervisors, roles 9
support
  ongoing 29
  partnerships 96–8
  peer 93–6
  seeking 126, 131–3
  see also stress management
SWOT analysis 83–4

teams
  roles 97
  working in 97
theorists, learning style 120
threats analysis 83–4
three brains exercise 120
time management 121–6
time, protected 104
training
  basic 20–1
  end-of-training interview 21
  mentees 22
  mentoring schemes 21–2
  potential mentors 21–2
  programmes, mentee 149
  programmes, mentor 145–9
transactional leaders 103
transformational leaders 103–4
trust, building 51–2

victims, Karpman triangle 113–15

weaknesses analysis 83–4
work flow control, time management
      122
work practice, development 98–104
working environment,
      health/safety/security 77–9